Everyday Miracles

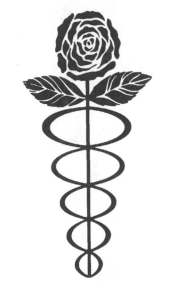

Homeopathy
in Action

Everyday Miracles

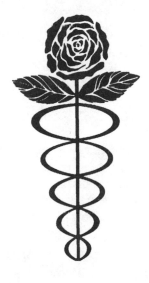

Homeopathy
in Action

Linda Johnston MD, DHt

Christine Kent Agency
Van Nuys, California

Everyday Miracles
Homeopathy in Action

ISBN: 1-877-691-00-3

Christine Kent Agency
17216 Saticoy # 348
Van Nuys, California 91406

Cover Design: Linda Johnston, MD and Yvonne Steinman
Illustrations: Yvonne Steinman
Graphs and Charts: Linda Johnston, MD

Published in the United States of America
10 9 8 7 6 5 4 3

To Samuel Hahnemann, MD

ACKNOWLEDGMENTS

To Judith Smith, MS, for her energetic, consistent support for this and all my projects. As my editor, her efforts brought this book to its present form. She has given me a new appreciation for the phrase "without whom this book never would have been published", for indeed, that is the case.

To George Vithoulkas whose dedication, brilliance and ceaseless work for Homeopathy has been the beacon of light guiding a new generation of Homeopaths. His confidence in me and encouragement have been a constant source of inspiration. He has shown me what is truly possible with Homeopathy, setting a standard to which I will always aspire.

To Alfons Geukens, MD whose mastery, skill and thorough understanding of the clinical application of Homeopathy has taught me what it means to be an excellent Homeopath. His dynamic teaching style and his energic and enthusiastic devotion to Homeopathy has served as a role model. I am grateful for his personal interest in my education.

To Thomas Marchioro, MD whose honor, integrity and caring commitment to each and every one of his patients taught me how to be a *real* doctor as a way of being, which rises above all else.

To Gilbert Denys of Homeoden Homeopathic Pharmacy for his friendship and commitment to the finest quality in Homeopathy and in the manufacture of Homeopathic remedies.

To Yvonne Steinman whose talent and artistry produced the illustrations for this book. She has the great gift of turning my ideas into pictures.

Acknowledgment goes to each and every one of my patients who are the real teachers for any doctor.

I also extend my appreciation to the following people for their friendship, encouragement, personal and professional support: John Switzer, MD; Guy Kokelenberg, MD; Roger van Zandvoort; Fernand Debats, MD; Durr Elmore, ND, DC; Misha Norland; Deitrich Grunow, MD; Volker Rohleder, MD; Henk van Hootcgcm, MD; Louis Klein, S Hom; K. S. Srinivasan, MD; Robert Rosscr, MD; Alize Timmerman; Andy Linial, DC; Patricia Ashley, MD; Terry Jacobs; John Taylor; Eric Anbergen; Frederic Schroyens; Kai Kroger; LaUna Huffines; Sanaya Roman; David Warkentin; Geraldine Saunders; Arthur Andrews; Sidney Omarr, John Swaney; John Enright, PhD; Tony and Marilee Hyman; Sctt Underwood; Norman and Eleanor Cousins; Henry J. Heimlich, MD; Jane Heimlich; Susan Krzywicki; Yvette Leten; Wane Ru and his entire staff; Steve Gordon, Esq; Patrick Andrews; Epi van de Pol; my father, Gerald F. Johnston, and my three wonderful brothers, Michael C. Johnston, Esq.; Scott G. Johnston and Bruce W. Johnston.

CONTENTS

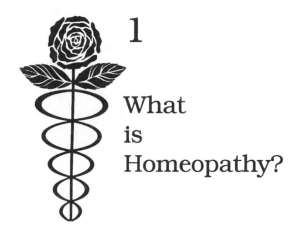

1
What
is
Homeopathy?

"Can you get rid of these?" Gladys, a very active and alert 91 year old woman, was pointing to her ankles. They had very large sores that hadn't healed in months. "My great grand daughter is getting married in six months and I want to look really nice that day. I want you to fix these ankles so I can wear nylon stockings and my best dress that comes just below my knees." I had my assignment loud and clear, so I began treatment immediately. No other treatment had helped Gladys at all. I know from experience how difficult it is to make any improvement in varicose ulcers as severe as hers, let alone completely heal them. This is especially true when there is poor circulation as is often the case in the elderly.

Eight months later, we were looking at the wedding pictures Gladys had brought to my office. She was radiant in her best dress and nylons, showing off her ankles. They were completely healed! My guess is that she stole the show that day!

✳ ✳ ✳

An attractive young mother came into my office. She certainly appeared healthy. Looking more closely, I could see that she was hiding her tears well. She had just come from the library where she had read everything she could find on multiple sclerosis. "At least now I know I'm not going crazy. As horrifying as this disease is, I would rather know what is going on. Finally this thing has a name." She had been suffering for over four years with weakness, blurred vision, difficulty concentrating and forgetfulness. She could recall having some of these symptoms as far back as 15 years ago. Now her vision was much worse and she could barely walk. The only way she could climb stairs was by pulling herself up the banister. She was extremely worried about being able to care for her family.

Four months after treatment, she was playing racquet ball and riding her exercise bike at least three times a week. Her visual problems had disappeared, her mind had become clear and her physical strength had improved. "My other doctors thought I'd be in a wheel chair by now. When I told them about my incredible improvement, they said I was probably just having a remission that would end soon. They told me remissions are common with multiple sclerosis but I've never had one before. I've just been getting steadily worse for 15 years. Why would I get a remission now, right after starting this treatment?"

❋ ❋ ❋

"Measles, definitely measles" I told 2 year old Thomas's mother. He had the fever, irritability and the characteristic rash. I gave a medication and his mother took him home to recover, expecting to wait out the normal 7 - 10 day course of the disease. She had been surprised when I asked her to call me the next day to let me know how he was doing.

When Thomas's mom called me with a progress report she

sounded a bit irritated. "I think you must have misdiagnosed my son. What other explanation is there for the fact that his rash is gone and so are all his other symptoms?"

✳ ✳ ✳

"It's all I can do to get dressed in the morning. I have excruciating pain every time I try to raise my arm. I'm in constant pain but the motion just makes it worse." Patricia was first diagnosed with arthritis 7 years ago. I had seen her shoulder x-ray and there was considerable joint destruction. It was no wonder she could barely move her arm.

Three months after treatment, she walked into my office in tears. I was very concerned until she said, "Today, for the first time in 7 years, I washed my own hair!" All her shoulder pain was gone and her mobility had increased remarkably. I ordered a repeat x-ray thinking that my treatment must have somehow reversed the joint destruction. How else could she have shown so much improvement? Amazingly, this x-ray looked just as bad as the first one.

✳ ✳ ✳

Twenty month old Jerry was always falling, tripping and running into things. This morning he fell off the front porch and almost cut off the tip of his little finger. When I first saw him there was blood everywhere. I thought he must have had an enormous accident. When I examined his finger tip, it was that dusky, dark color which strikes fear in a doctor's heart because it means the finger tip won't survive. I gave him an emergency medication. Right before our eyes, the bleeding stopped and the finger turned a healthy, bright pink again. To finish the job, I could have put a few stitches in the wound myself but it had been such a bad injury, I thought I would ask a surgeon to do it.

Surprised at the good condition of such a deep wound, the surgeon asked Jerry's mom how she had stopped the bleeding but changed the subject before she could tell him. I had given Jerry 5¢ worth of medicine, the surgeon's bill was over $900.

To some these might seem like Miracles, in my practice they happen Everyday.

Many of us have observed things about health and medicine that just don't seem to make sense. Why do some people live to be 90 and do so many things we all know are bad for us, while other people get sick even though they exercise and really watch what they eat? Why do some people always have so much energy while others can barely make it through the day? How come several people in the same office always get every cold that's going around, yet there are one or two others that never seem to get sick? Modern medicine just doesn't seem to have good answers for these kinds of questions.

The type of medicine that has grown to dominance in America in the last 40-50 years is proud to be the master of medical technology and technique. Sadly, all this expertise has not made it the master of health. We still have a vast array of both acute and chronic illnesses. In addition, there is the tremendous expense of maintaining the current health care delivery system. Despite the limitations, problems and costs of modern medicine, many have not yet discovered an adequate alternative.

Naturally, everyone wants the very best medical care for themselves and their families. The desire for good health is not new. Today the difference is many people are seeking answers and medical treatment outside of that offered by the conventional medical establishment. If any other medical treatment is to be used, it must be an effective, safe and legitimate treatment administered by a skilled physician or practitioner. How can you know what is legitimate and truly effective and what is not?

What if I told you that there is a system of medical treatment that could answer the questions we've just asked and others you may have? A system that:

• is based on sound scientific principles.
• has a long history of consistent, reliable results and real cures.
• is safe, affordable, effective, and without toxic drugs or side effects.
• ultimately allows you to become free of the need to receive medical care.

Would you want to know more? I did too!

From the time I was 14, I wanted to be a doctor. I would read everything about medical history and notable medical people I could get my hands on. I wanted to join the ranks of those who had been dedicated to the improvement of the human condition, and to carry on, in my own small way, the work to which they had contributed so greatly.

Clearly knowing what I wanted to do in life, I raced through college and medical school. Then, during the clinical portion of both medical school and post graduate training, I became overwhelmed by the magnitude of the problems and misery I saw. I was also disheartened because there seemed so little I could do to help, despite all that modern medicine offered.

Slowly, my perspective changed. I began to see the same kinds of problems I had read about in my history books: issues of care, compassion, understanding, suffering, economics, politics, ignorance and integrity.

I began to recognize the limitations of modern medical thought and practices for making real changes in people's lives.

After all that I had seen in training, the only aspect of medicine that still held promise for me was establishing my own private practice where I could do things differently. I might not be able to change the whole medical system, but I could keep my little corner the way I wanted it for the benefit of my patients.

After starting my practice, I was absorbed by the business of medicine. The transition from the academic environment to the "real world" required a whole new realm of skills. I was learning to apply the medical knowledge I had gained in training to the business of private practice.

During this time, I noticed some things I hadn't learned in medical school. I began to see certain trends in my patients. Many people just weren't getting any better, in fact, the more "medicine" I did for them the worse they became. They didn't want my fancy knowledge; they wanted compassion, understanding and a generous dose of common sense. They wanted to feel better, not just in their flesh and bones, but on the inside, in their hearts and spirits.

There I was, armed with all the best that modern medicine could give them and it still wasn't enough. Maybe it just wasn't enough of the right thing. I didn't know. The only thing I did know was that I had to do something differently. I had thought that having my own private practice would have been enough to make things different for my patients. In fact, nothing much had changed at all. I knew I had to supplement my medical knowledge with something else to attend to these unsolved problems and the human side of my patients.

From my earlier studies, I knew that the ancient civilizations of Egypt, Greece, China, India and Tibet all had medical systems and many of those cultures were magnificent, prosperous and long lived. I decided to start investigating there. I studied herbal medicine, acupuncture, nutrition, ayurvedic medicine, yoga and other healing methods and my medical practice began to evolve.

It wasn't that I had changed much of
what I was DOING
for diagnosis and treatment;
I had changed the way
I was THINKING
about health, illness and human beings.

I still didn't know how to go about providing medical care from this new orientation and incorporating it into the vast amount of benefit that was also available from modern medical practices. What could I do, *today,* to help the lines of people filing through my office with rashes, infections, depressions, anxieties or any one of a thousand other ailments?

I came upon the answer to this question quite by accident; I literally stumbled upon it. While visiting a long-time friend, I hit my knee cap on her coffee table. I had a lot of pain and a nasty bruise was quickly forming. My friend offered me a Homeopathic remedy. I only accepted the remedy because I totally trusted her. Besides, those two little pellets looked like they couldn't cause any harm, or do any good for that matter! The pain subsided quickly and I forgot the whole thing. Several hours later I looked at my knees. To my surprise, the bruise was *gone!* I couldn't even tell which knee had been injured. There wasn't any abrasion, swelling or pain! Everyone knows that a forceful bump causes a bruise and that bruises take more than a week to go away. Yet my bruise and all my symptoms were gone in just a few hours! What I experienced could not be explained by conventional medicine, and yet I couldn't just ignore what had happened. Medicine, as I had known it, was about to undergo an enormous change.

Naturally I was skeptical about Homeopathy at first, but as I investigated further, my skepticism turned to amazement.

The rest is simply a story of my continuing involvement in Homeopathy through study, classes, seminars, reading, research, lecturing, teaching, writing and treating patients.

*I am enthusiastic about
the science of Homeopathy
because IT WORKS.*

Homeopathy is a scientific and holistic system of medicine developed 200 years ago by Samuel Hahnemann, a German physician. It works to release people from the bonds of illness that have crippled them for so very long; restoring them to vibrant health.

What exactly is Homeopathy and how does it work? How can it cure diseases that have baffled the best of modern medicine and do so with non-toxic, safe medications given for only short periods of time? Homeopathy cures disease by naturally activating and boosting the body's own inner ability for healing and self-cure.

*Homeopathy creates
a very deep and profound healing
that most doctors have never seen
and most patients have never experienced.*

This is what can be expected when the enormous capacity of the human being for self-healing is released, activated and allowed to progress.

Homeopathic medicines, called remedies, act deeply in the body to stimulate those built-in mechanisms of self healing. A remedy is needed when these systems lack enough of their own power to eliminate a disease completely and restore health. With the extra activation that a Homeopathic remedy provides, the body can shed the symptoms that resulted from the disease. Dramatic and long lasting improvement or cure is seen in a wide variety of illnesses, many of which have been called chronic or incurable.

There are no long-term medications, restrictive diets, counseling or psycho-therapy with Homeopathic treatment. There is just plain and effective prescribing of the correct, non-toxic Homeopathic remedy to cure the disease and restore vitality and health.

The principles of Homeopathy are based on natural law. Diseases and the way symptoms develop follow the same laws of physics, biology, physiology and Nature that all other events in life *must* obey. Homeopathy provides a complete framework for understanding the predictable and orderly way that the human being maintains health and responds to illness. By reading this book, you will gain this understanding. Many unexplained and puzzling aspects of medicine and health will become very clear to you. As so many of my patients, students and those I have lectured say, "Homeopathy just makes so much sense!"

Homeopathy uses only plants, minerals and a few animal products as the sources for its remedies. These substances are gathered from nature and processed in a special way that is unique to Homeopathy. This processing technique eliminates the toxic properties of a substance while retaining its deep healing qualities.   By using medicines prepared this way, Homeopathy can safely use plants or minerals that may be harmful or toxic if used in their natural form.

Homeopathy is the third most commonly prescribed form of medical treatment worldwide. In America, Samuel Hahnemann is the only medical doctor with a statue and monument in Washington, D.C.

The form of Homeopathy practiced today that most closely

adheres to the original work of Dr. Hahnemann is called Classical Homeopathy. It follows very specific rules and is a precise, detailed and accurate method of prescribing Homeopathic remedies. Classical Homeopathy has three main aspects:

1. Using specially prepared Homeopathic remedies.
2. Using symptoms to prescribe the remedy by the Law of Similars.
3. Prescribing only one remedy at a time and allowing it to complete its action before giving another.

All three of these requirements must be met for a treatment to be truly called Homeopathic Medicine. We will talk more about these three requirements in the following chapters.

Other methods of prescribing and using remedies have often been done in the name of Homeopathy. I have found the original, Classical Homeopathy as developed by Dr. Samuel Hahnemann, to be the most accurate and effective method. Other methods have not resulted in the long term benefit by curing the serious, complex and chronic diseases that Classical Homeopathy is known to cure.

Reading this book will provide you with a foundation of knowledge and a complete enough understanding of the principles of Classical Homeopathy to make your own evaluation.

The science of Homeopathy is a complete medical system that can treat acute illnesses as well as improve and cure many chronic illnesses that plague our society. The only limitation to Homeopathy is the way it is performed or applied by individual doctors and practitioners. Similarly, music may bring great joy, peace and tranquility to the listener. If the music is unpleasant or amateurish, do we condemn the entire art of music or merely the performer or composer?

In the hands of a qualified, knowledgeable physician or practitioner, and judged on its merits and results alone, Classical Homeopathy consistently provides the miraculous, safe and wonderful healing capacities that have been demon-strated for two centuries.

Many people first experience or witness the benefits of Homeopathic treatment by taking remedies themselves or by giving them to their family members. It is easy to learn to use these non-prescription remedies to treat minor accidents, injuries, colds, flus and other acute illnesses quickly and successfully. Many doctors practicing Homeopathy today, myself included, are doing so because we have personally experienced dramatic cures using Homeopathic remedies to treat these types of illnesses.

The term "Holistic Medicine" is familiar to many people and I am often asked if it is the same as Homeopathy. The two are related but are not exactly the same.

Holistic Medicine is a philosophy; Homeopathy is a medical system.

The holistic philosophy in medicine states that a person is one unified being and everything about them affects their health. The foods we eat, the way we sleep, our temperament, our reaction to stress, our character and life style are all just as important as the actual physical symptoms in the diagnosis and treatment of an illness. No separation can be made between physical symptoms and emotions. Every aspect is intertwined with all our other aspects. The holistic philosophy further asserts that any medical system that really hopes to improve a person's health *must* take all these factors into consideration. Any therapy can be "holistic" if it has and uses this philosophy.

Homeopathy is one of only a few legitimate medical systems that is truly holistic in thought and in practice. Acupuncture and Chiropractic are other fine examples of effective holistic medical systems. Homeopathy, Acupuncture and Chiropractic follow the idea of the unity of the human being.

The human being is an integrated system having three main aspects: physical, emotional and mental.

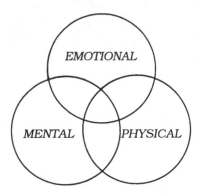

All three areas interact, influence and affect each other. It is not possible to determine our true health by looking only at one aspect. It is no more accurate to assume that you are totally healthy because your lungs work well than it is to think that your finances are in good order because you have a pocket full of money.

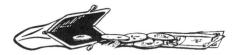

Every part needs to be considered in determining your total health, just as all your assets and liabilities need to be counted to understand your complete financial picture.

With conventional medical treatment, when a particular symptom goes away the patient is declared to be cured and restored to health. Often the disappearance of a symptom or even a group of symptoms may cause a decrease in overall health. The holistic philosophy requires that all areas be evaluated both before treatment and again after treatment. A cure only takes place when all aspects of the person improve as compared to the first assessment.

Perhaps I can illustrate this by using an example. Let's say that you go to a conventional doctor seeking medical treatment for a stomach ache with acid indigestion. He gives you a medication to stop these symptoms, which it does very well. Because the medication can adversely effect your liver, the doctor says that you now must return every two months to have a blood test to be sure your liver is functioning properly. Later you notice that you aren't sleeping as well due to some occasional stiffness in your joints. If we just look at your stomach problem, it would appear that you have been cured, but what about your disturbed sleep and the potential effects on your liver?

Conventional medicine is symptom specific, Homeopathy is person specific.

In evaluating results and determining cure, the holistic approach looks at you as a whole. It looks at all your symptoms including any changes and effects you have after treatment, not just the condition of your stomach. Though your stomach may be better, new problems in other areas have occurred as a result of the treatment. From the holistic perspective, you may actually be worse off now than you were with your stomach ache!

Thus, the term "holistic" is a philosophy that looks at each of us as a complex, integrated system that includes all aspects of the physical body, the emotions and the mind. As a foundation for Homeopathy, this philosophy and its principles are used both in diagnosis and treatment. Homeopathy demands that the total of all areas of the patient must be improved to call the patient cured.

This is a fundamental difference between Homeopathy and the dominant, conventional medical system in the world today, frequently called Allopathic medicine. Allopathic medicine does not have a holistic view and, of course, Homeopathy does. There are many other important differences between the two such as: what constitutes health, how diseases develop, and the meaning and importance of symptoms. These differences have a major impact on the effectiveness of each medical system and on the overall health of the patients treated.

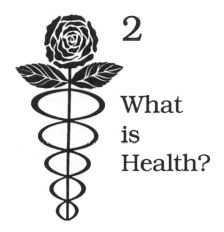

2

What
is
Health?

Ah, HEALTH! Health clubs, health foods, health spas, health maintenance organizations. "I want to be healthier!" "How can I regain my health?" "I just don't feel very healthy. I've already improved my diet and started exercising. Isn't there anything else I can do to feel really good again?" "Is declining health all I have to look forward to as I get older? Is there something I can do to make sure my mind stays sharp and my body stays in good shape?"

People from all over the country are asking me questions like these about how they can be as healthy as possible. These are not just the "heath conscious", but individuals from a wide range of ages, life styles, social circumstances, educational backgrounds and professions.

Health is something we all want, yet what exactly are we seeking? Unless we know what we're looking for, how will we know when we find it? We all know when we don't feel well, but can we clearly define the qualities that make us healthy?

A clear definition of health is especially important when evaluating medical treatment designed to achieve health. How are you going to know if the treatment you're receiving is improving your health? How will you know if a treatment today will cause problems in the future or when to stop because it's done all that it can?

It may surprise you to know that I, like most other doctors, went through four years of medical school without once being given a real definition of health. I was taught that I must help patients achieve health, but I was never given any yardstick by which to measure that achievement. I learned about diseases, physical symptoms and pathological processes, but not about health. The focus of all this training was almost exclusively on the physical aspect of a person, while excluding emotional and mental health. Was health then to be defined only in terms of the physical body? Obviously, not!

So that we may reach our goal of health, we will need a comprehensive, dynamic definition of *health* that is applicable to the *whole* person and to all situations.

Let's start with the expert. Webster and his New Universal Unabridged Dictionary states that Health is "physical and mental well-being, normality of mental and physical functions". This definition does meet our requirement of including the whole person, however, the terms "well-being" and "normality" are just as vague as the term "health".

Webster then goes on to say that health is "freedom from defect, pain or disease", defining health by what it is not, rather than what it is. Defining health in terms of a lack of disease, pain or disability, implies that by eliminating these conditions we will restore health. This is simply not so. That is similar to stating that we are financially secure if we are not in debt. Paying off all our debts would only give us financial relief, not financial security. The mere absence of debt compared to all the possibilities there are with an abundance of money is similar to the difference between the absence of disease and experiencing true health.

True health
must be thought of in positive, dynamic terms,
not simply as the absence of disease.

In addition to using positive and dynamic terms, our definition of health must encompass every aspect of the whole functioning human being, including the emotional and mental areas as well as the physical. By using this definition, both you as a patient and your doctor must be able to assess your overall state of health. The definition must, therefore, contain specific goals and criteria so that you will both know whether you are moving toward the state of health or away from it into a deeper disease state. Let's look now at a new, expanded definition that takes these ideas into consideration:

Health is freedom on the physical level. Our bodies perform all the functions and tasks for which they were designed, with ease, grace and energy. Each part of the body, from the cells to the organ systems, operates in an integrated and harmonious way for optimum efficiency allowing us to respond quickly and appropriately to situations arising in our environment. Our bodies function automatically without any problems or limitations that call attention to themselves through symptoms or pain.

Health is freedom on the emotional level. We experience the wide array of emotions possible in a positive and enriching way. We have joyful, satisfying relationships with family, friends, society and ourselves. We can express and receive love freely and make deep, fulfilling relationships with others. Our desires are balanced and moderate. We show concern and consideration for the welfare of others. We can fully appreciate beauty and Nature.

Health is freedom on the mental level. We experience positive, creative self-expression through a career, service or art. The various functions of the mind operate with clarity and efficiency. Personal ideas, thoughts, concepts and imagination are turned into positive and meaningful actions. True mental health also includes our innate desire to be of service to other people, to society and to the world.

Using this broad and encompassing definition of health we now have a yardstick by which we can measure our own health. Do you meet all the requirements listed? Are you as healthy as you would like to be? Do you experience the kind of freedom inherent in true health? Is your medical treatment successfully restoring your health?

We now have an effective way to evaluate any medical treatment. We can look at the whole person and can provide what is needed, when and where it is needed. Most importantly, this new definition of health provides a perspective on the enormous and magnificent potential inherent in each and every one of us.

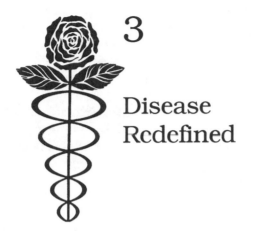

3

Disease
Redefined

Now that we have a new way of looking at health, we also need a new way of thinking about disease.

We usually refer to a disease by the name we give to a collection of symptoms. It's a short-hand notation summarizing all the symptoms that are present in a particular condition. If someone says he has allergies, hypertension, depression or arthritis, he assumes that you will know what specific symptoms he has. Is this really the case? Does that disease name convey his exact experience and all his symptoms?

Let's use arthritis as an example. The term "arthritis" is given to a group of symptoms including, but not limited to, pain, swelling, stiffness and inflammation of any joint or group of joints. Far from having a single set of similar symptoms, there are tremendous differences, as any group of arthritis sufferers could tell you. Some have stiffness in the morning, some in the evening, some have pain that is worse in cold weather while others are better in the cold. Some have pains that stay in certain joints and some have pains that wander around. Some have red, hot, swollen joints and others have deformed joints.

There are no characteristic symptoms for the disease called "arthritis". If we look at all the different symptoms that define the disease, including individual patient experiences of these symptoms there are hundreds, if not thousands of different forms of arthritis. Yet we call these vastly different forms by one term: arthritis. With such great variety, is it really possible to say these are all the same disease?

Of course, there are sub-categories of arthritis that include rheumatoid, degenerative and osteoarthritis. There is great overlapping in the kinds of symptoms for each of these types of arthritis. As is usually the case, the sub-categories of a disease have very little or no relationship to the specific symptoms of the patient.

All the familiar disease names are terms representing collections of a variety of symptoms. Headache, indigestion, sciatica, backache, depression, flu, asthma and hypoglycemia are just a few examples. Anyone labeled with a disease name most often doesn't have all the symptoms associated with that disease. One study investigating Premenstrual Syndrome collected over 500 different symptoms reported by women suffering from this problem, yet each woman only experienced a few of that number at any given time. Even disease types that might be assumed to be very specific, such as multiple sclerosis, angina, high blood pressure or strep throat each consist of a variety of symptoms and individual patient experiences.

This grouping of symptoms into disease categories evolved to help make diagnoses and treat patients. Rarely, if ever, are the details of individual symptoms or experiences used or needed by conventional medical doctors. For example, a particular medicine is prescribed for arthritis, regardless of the location of the pain, whether it is worse at a specific time of day or has any other distinguishing characteristics. Generally, there is one treatment and one therapeutic approach for everyone who has been labeled with a given disease name.

*The conventional medical system strives
to standardize all treatment
with the goal of eliminating
individual differences.*

This process of standardizing has even extended to Medicare payments for treatment of patients. Medicare pays a predetermined, fixed amount for each hospitalization and treatment of a disease category. It is the job of the doctors and hospitals to fit the patient into one of those disease categories so they will receive payment. There is little or no financial provision for variety, severity or individual needs for treatment. This is the extent to which government and modern medicine has come in its efforts to homogenize and standardize the infinite variety of human illnesses and diseases into limited and convenient categories.

The flaw in all this is that the disease name is not the actual disease, it is only a convenient label representing a collection of symptoms. There are no characteristic symptoms for everyone. Does this mean that each person with his individual collection of symptoms has a different disease? How can we possibly understand and treat disease with such diversity? Is there a common thread? How can all this be unified and still encompass this diversity?

To do this we must look at disease from a new perspective. Let's start with the symptoms, the only tangible evidence available that a disease is really present. We are so accustomed to common disease names that it is often difficult to think only in terms of symptoms.

Beginning with a patient's actual symptoms, it should be possible to understand the nature of his disease. Let's use our example of arthritis to see if this is true.

A patient is told he has arthritis.

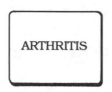

We know by the name "arthritis" that the problem is in the joints but the name doesn't tell us the patient's exact symptoms. Let's say he has stiffness, pain and swelling in the knee joints. Our search for the nature of the arthritis begins by asking, "What caused those specific symptoms?" In other words, what pathway does it take?

ARTHRITIS

↖

?

Medical science tells us that damaged cartilage in the joint is causing the symptoms.

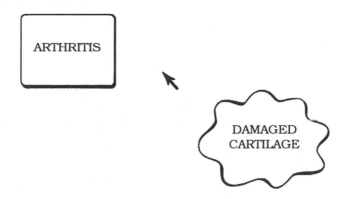

There is some debris in the joint and the joint surfaces have become roughened. They can't slide easily over each other anymore. It is understandable why the knee joints are so painful, stiff and swollen. Is this the cause of his problems?

No, this condition doesn't just happen to everyone. What caused this damage to occur at all?

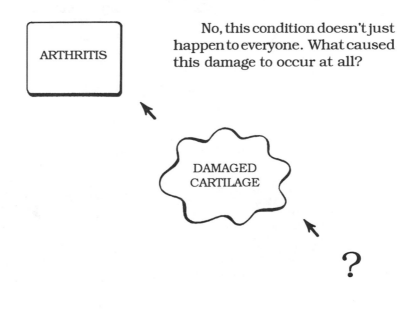

The damage to the cartilage was caused by inflammation in the knee joint.

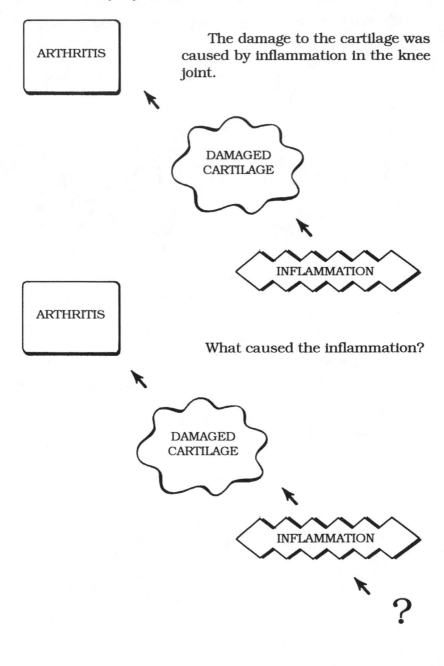

What caused the inflammation?

It could have been caused by an injury, but often in cases with these symptoms there hasn't been any injury to the joint. The cause of the inflammation is the release of certain chemicals into the joint.

These chemical factors initiate the inflammation which then produces the damage that causes the symptoms.

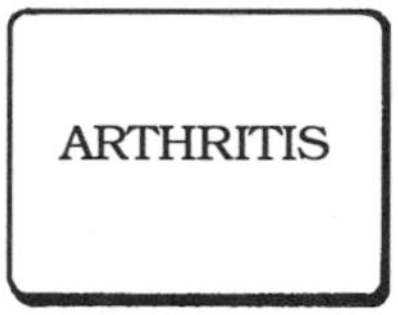

ARTHRITIS

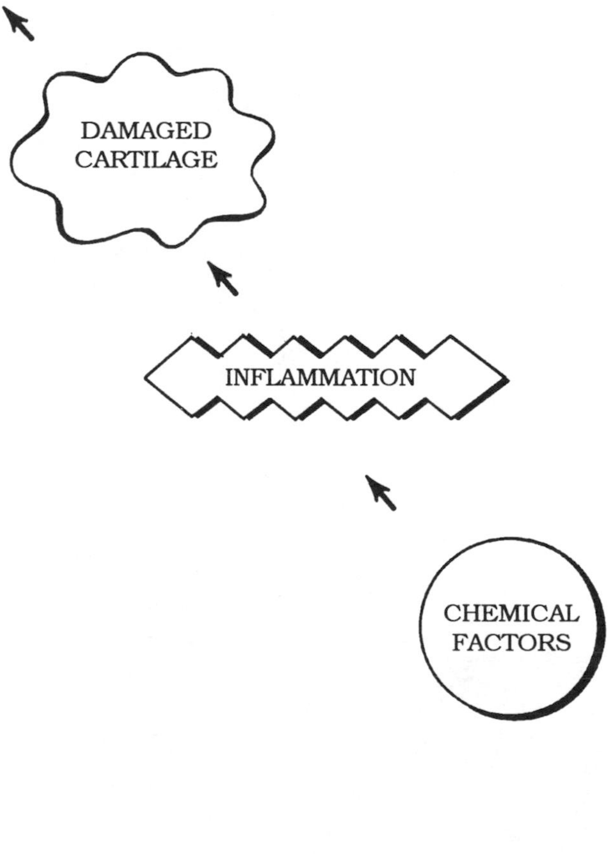

DAMAGED CARTILAGE

INFLAMMATION

CHEMICAL FACTORS

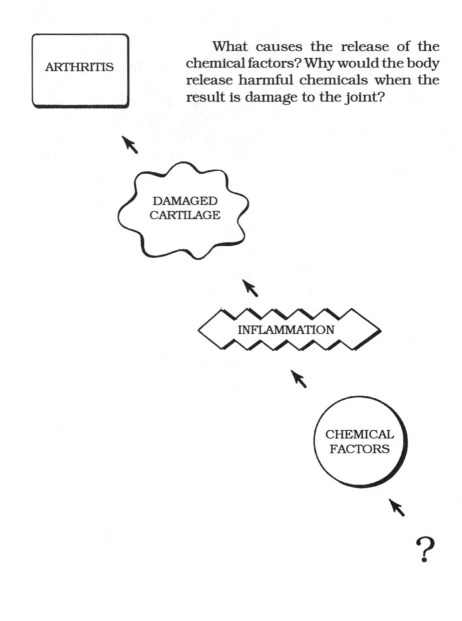

ARTHRITIS

What causes the release of the chemical factors? Why would the body release harmful chemicals when the result is damage to the joint?

DAMAGED CARTILAGE

INFLAMMATION

CHEMICAL FACTORS

?

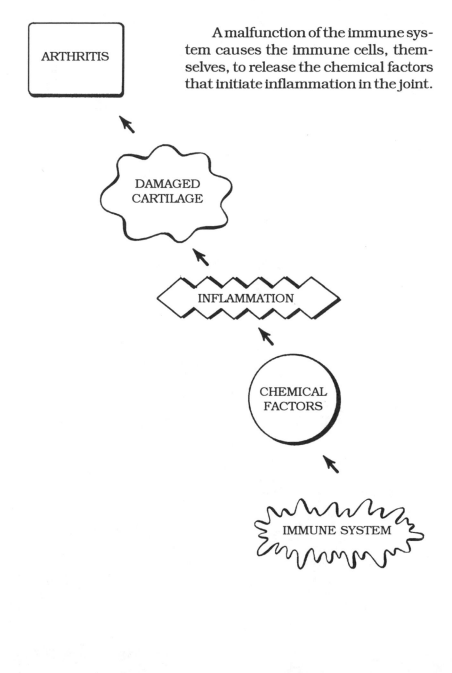

A malfunction of the immune system causes the immune cells, themselves, to release the chemical factors that initiate inflammation in the joint.

What causes the immune system to malfunction in the first place? The answer is, we just don't know!

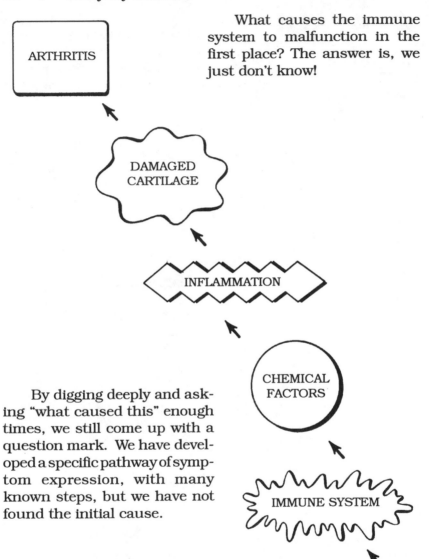

By digging deeply and asking "what caused this" enough times, we still come up with a question mark. We have developed a specific pathway of symptom expression, with many known steps, but we have not found the initial cause.

Let's look at another common problem, high blood pressure. As the name suggests, blood pressure is the amount of pressure inside the blood vessels.

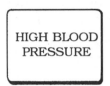

We begin again by asking what caused the blood pressure to be elevated.

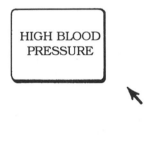

Arteriosclerosis or "hardening of the arteries" is a common cause.

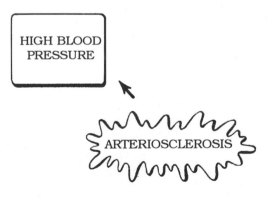

The arteries become "hardened" when the resilient elastic tissue of the artery wall is replaced by other tissues and substances that are not elastic such as scar, cholesterol, and collagen. This loss of flexibility and elasticity results in a narrow, contracted artery that, in turn, results in increased pressure inside the artery.

What causes this hardening process to start? How does the normal artery turn into the "lead pipe" of arteriosclerosis?

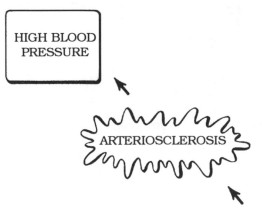

?

This process starts with a little bit of damage, small rips and tears, in the lining of the artery. As in other injuries, scar tissue forms as the body does its best to repair itself.

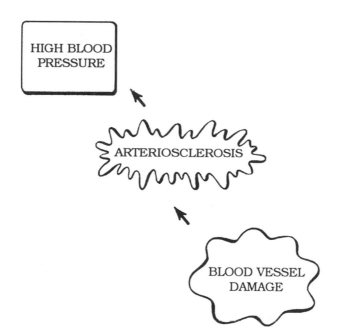

Originally, the lining of the blood vessel was very smooth, allowing blood to flow easily. With scar tissue in the lining of the artery, the blood can't flow in such an even and perfect way. There is a small amount of turbulence causing the blood to hit the artery walls. This greater strain results in further damage to the artery's lining, more rips and tears. As the body repairs this damage more scar tissue, cholesterol deposits, and other materials are formed. This continues to accumulate over time and results in a thickened, severely damaged artery. This is called arteriosclerosis.

Medical science knows a lot about these stages in the development of arteriosclerosis. The next step is to ask why the small rips occur? What causes the initial damage?

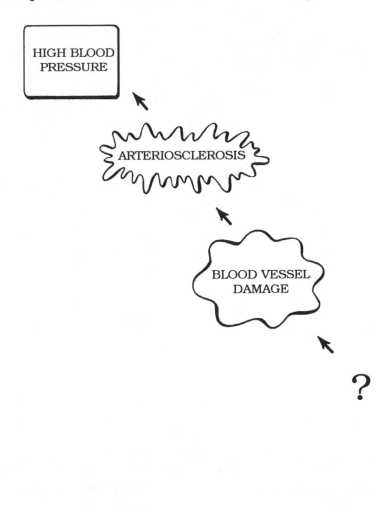

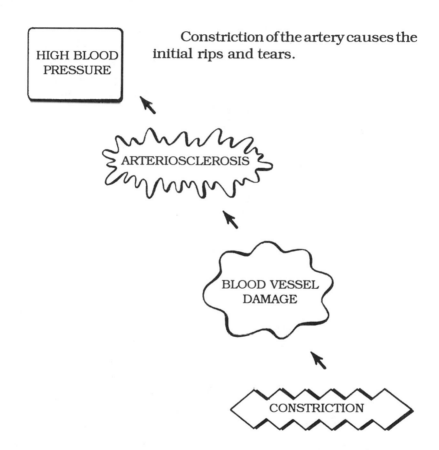

HIGH BLOOD PRESSURE

Constriction of the artery causes the initial rips and tears.

ARTERIOSCLEROSIS

BLOOD VESSEL DAMAGE

CONSTRICTION

There are many circumstances in which it is normal and healthy for the arteries to constrict. Fright, exercise, and experiencing certain emotions are just a few examples. These and other stressful situations cause a normal physiological reaction of the body known as the "stress response" that prepares and protects us from impending danger.

A constant level of stress, however, causes the "stress response" with its normal body changes, to be active continually. This unrelenting onslaught of changes in the body that are designed to occur intermittently causes great harm. While well tolerated on the short term basis, permanent constriction of the arteries results in damage to the artery's lining.

What keeps the "stress response" active?

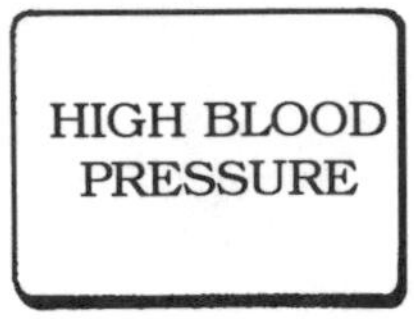

HIGH BLOOD PRESSURE

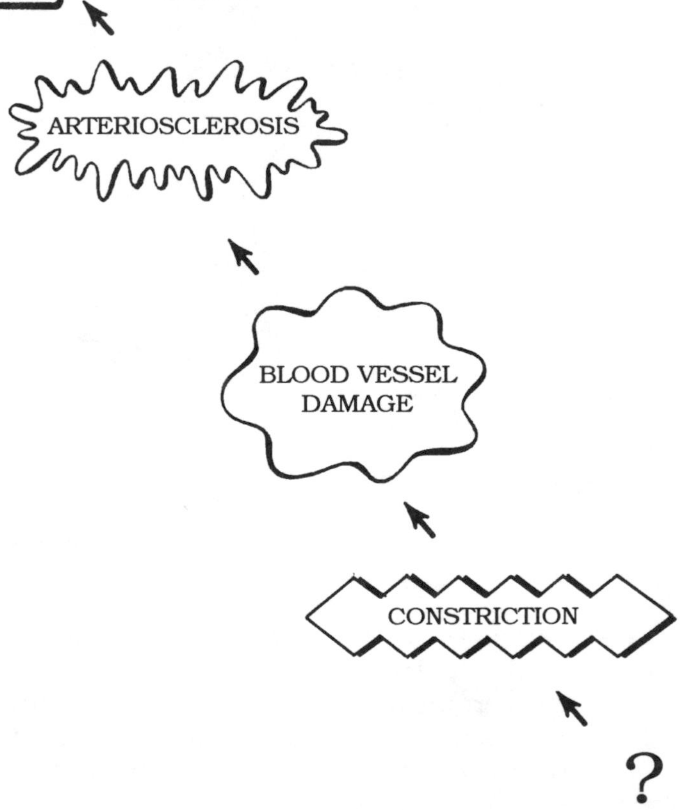

ARTERIOSCLEROSIS

BLOOD VESSEL DAMAGE

CONSTRICTION

?

Continual stress is the primary cause of the constriction that eventually results in arteriosclerosis and high blood pressure.

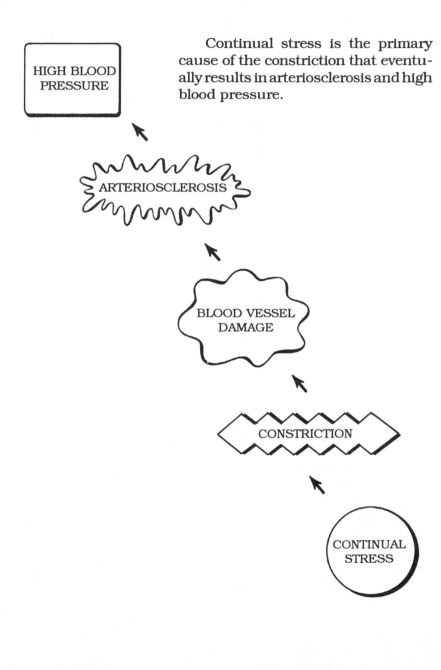

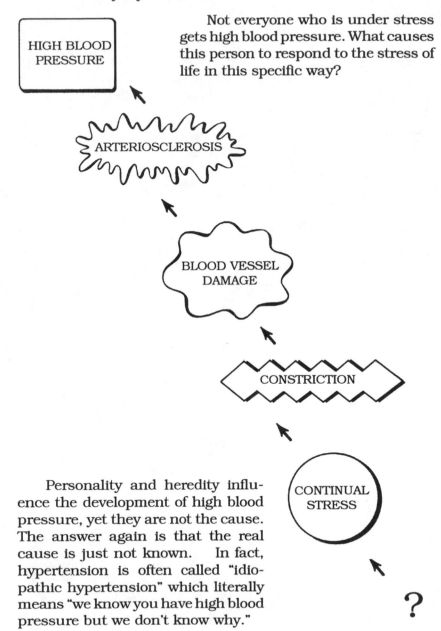

Not everyone who is under stress gets high blood pressure. What causes this person to respond to the stress of life in this specific way?

Personality and heredity influence the development of high blood pressure, yet they are not the cause. The answer again is that the real cause is just not known. In fact, hypertension is often called "idiopathic hypertension" which literally means "we know you have high blood pressure but we don't know why."

Any disease process or collection of symptoms follows the same pattern that we just established for arthritis and high blood pressure. We know many mechanical steps in symptom development but not the actual initiating cause. The true cause of any set of symptoms is represented by the "?", all the rest is the effect of the initial cause.

We can now say that disease is not the collection of symptoms, it is the cause of the symptoms. The symptoms are not the definition of disease, they are the *results* of disease. This may seem a subtle difference, but it is a very important distinction.

Disease is the cause of Symptoms, Symptoms are the results of Disease.

Another way of understanding the difference between the cause and the symptoms in a disease is to examine how a slide projector works. A slide projector has a light source, a slide and a screen.

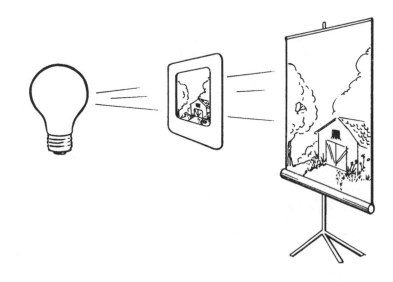

The light shines through the slide, producing a picture on the screen. The picture depends entirely upon what is on the slide. The slide is the cause and the picture is the effect. It isn't possible to change the picture by walking up to the screen and trying to move the tree to the left and the house to the right. You just can't do it! That is because the picture is only the effect. Changes can only be made at the level of the cause. To change the picture (effect) on the screen it is necessary to change the slide (cause).

The disease is the same as the slide and the patient's symptoms are the same as the picture on the screen. Just as the slide produces the picture on the screen, the disease (cause) produces the symptoms (effects) on the body.

Now, what practical application does this new definition of disease have? Does it help doctors do their job of taking care of patients?

Conventional medicine or any therapy which only treats the symptoms, is like going up to the screen and trying to make changes there. Homeopathy treats at the level of the cause, getting rid of the disease. Without the disease or cause, the symptoms can no longer exist. They just naturally and permanently disappear.

Modern medicine doesn't bother speculating about the unknown initiating cause of symptoms. Doctors usually want to know just enough to enable them to eliminate the symptoms. They do this by giving medications. In our example of arthritis, the doctor will prescribe a medicine that will stop the inflammation thereby reducing pain and damage to the joint.

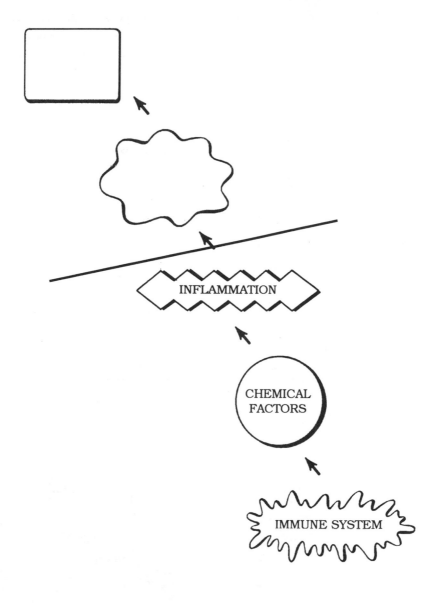

A medication for high blood pressure can force the body to stop constricting the arteries, thereby reducing the blood pressure.

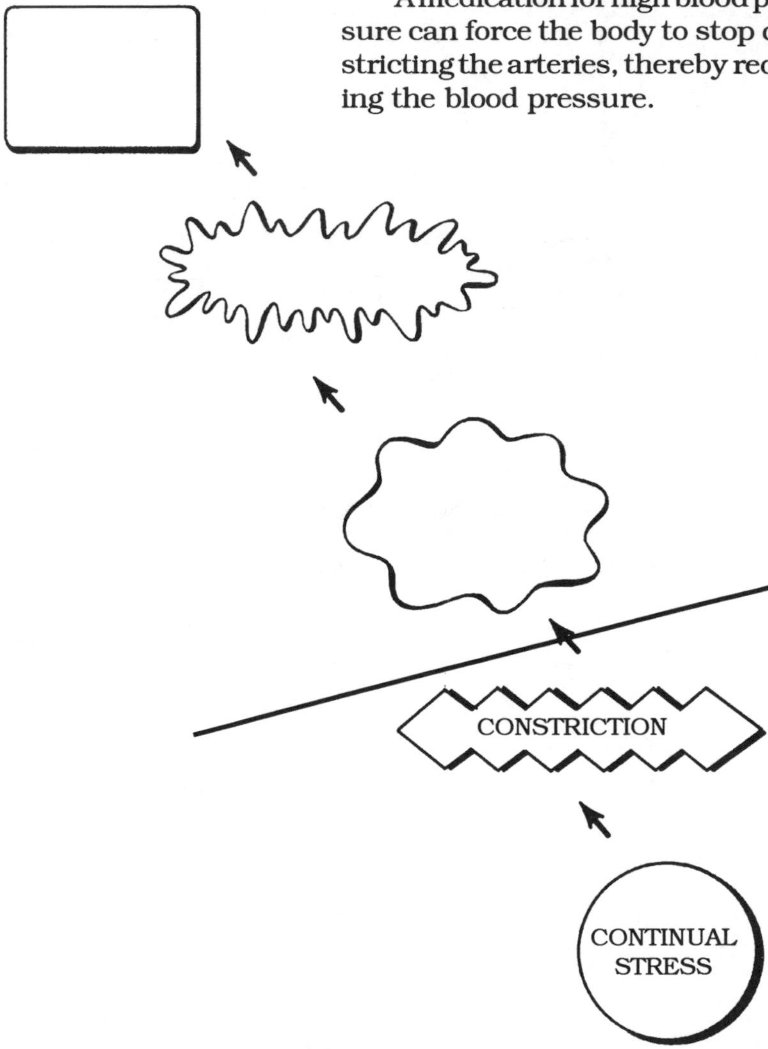

CONSTRICTION

CONTINUAL
STRESS

These efforts seem beneficial to the patient, however, the disease causing the symptoms has not been cured, it has only been blocked. The force behind the blocked disease pathway will find another outlet, another path to follow. Other symptoms will develop and the patient will continue in poor health.

Taking a medicine that blocks one step of the disease pathway without eliminating the cause creating it is similar to putting a dam across a river.

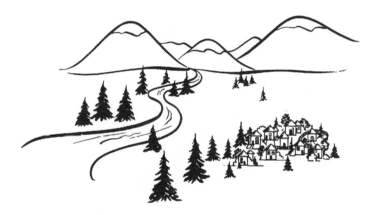

The dam stops the river from flowing along its normal course but it does not keep the river, itself, from flowing. Behind the dam, the water is becoming a very large force.

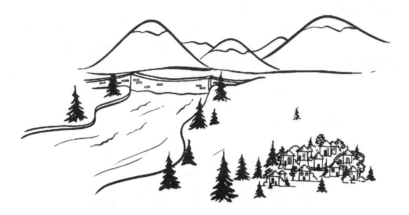

If this large force of water is not allowed to spill through the dam, then it will find other places to flow. Here, it flows into the surrounding forest and nearby town.

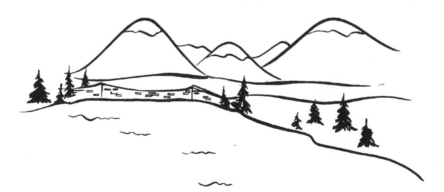

Obstructing the river like this is the same as giving medicine to prevent arthritic inflammation; it blocks a stage in the disease pathway. The medicine does nothing to stop or reduce the disease force which simply finds a new way of expressing itself through different symptoms. It is the continued presence of this disease which requires ongoing medications to stop the symptoms from returning in a chronic disease.

Homeopathy treats and eliminates the disease or cause. All the effects of the disease, the symptoms, then go away. This is why a short course of medication is all that is required with Homeopathic treatment.

We can now see why it is so important for us to understand the distinction between disease and symptoms if we are to achieve good health.

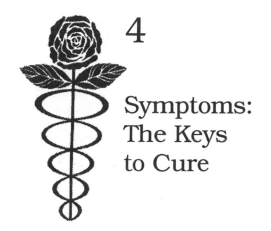

4

Symptoms:
The Keys
to Cure

Symptoms are the key to Homeopathic medicine. In chapter three we said that disease is the cause of all symptoms and therefore, all symptoms are the result of disease. Let's expand on these ideas to see what symptoms really are and how they can be used in the diagnosis and selection of the specific Homeopathic remedy that will cure the patient.

A symptom is any characteristic from any aspect of the whole human being. This includes all the complaints, problems or limitations from the emotions and mind as well as the body. Thoughts, reactions to stress or weather conditions, sleep patterns, temperament, food preferences, effects of childhood experiences, family, social and work experiences, emotional traumas or upsets and physical complaints are all examples of symptoms. Other symptoms might be a strong liking for salty foods, a preference for sleeping on your left side or waking up at three in the morning and falling back to sleep at four. These may all seem common place, but they provide very valuable information about each person as a unique individual. We call many things "normal" because we have never experienced life without them. They are actually symptoms representing our overall state of health.

There are thousands of these pieces of information about us. Many are used to determine our correct Homeopathic remedy. Not all of these, however, are symptoms of disease. Many are simply characteristics of us as unique individuals. To decide which of these are symptoms and which are personal characteristics we must again look at our new definition of health.

Health is a state of FREEDOM.

Any of our characteristics that prevent freedom are symptoms and will be eliminated through Homeopathic treatment. Those qualities that do not cause problems will remain and can be enhanced after treatment.

The process of collecting enough information from a patient to make the correct prescription can take up to two hours. It's often a pleasant surprise for patients new to Homeopathy to have the doctor give so much attention to them and their long ignored, unexplained and annoying symptoms.

Our bodies express themselves in many, many ways. Unfortunately, most people, including doctors, don't realize the importance of this information. This is a natural result of the tendency of conventional medicine to group symptoms together into a limited number of disease categories. Any information that falls outside what is required to assign a disease category is either ignored or simply goes unnoticed. A person might go to a doctor because he just isn't feeling well but when he tries to discuss his symptoms, sensations or emotions the doctor will overlook them because his symptoms don't fit into any disease category or diagnosis. Do you know anyone who has experienced this? Of course, we all do!

Homeopaths know that symptoms are the body "talking" in the only way it knows how. The disease can only be understood through the evidence given by the symptoms. This is why the

Homeopathic physician looks at all aspects and symptoms to understand the patient's disease. Looking at the symptoms, the Homeopathic physician will get a picture of the disease. Just as in our example of the slide projector, if we look closely at what is on the screen (symptoms), we also will know what is on the slide (disease).

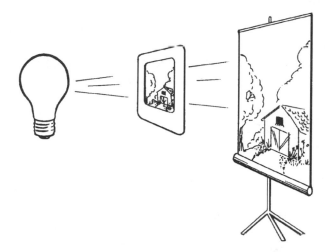

There is a commonly held belief that a disease can be lurking in a person's body without the knowledge of the body's owner. This mistaken idea is responsible for a tremendous amount of anxiety and fear concerning health issues. Who wouldn't be nervous thinking that a terrible disease could be growing quietly and maliciously inside us without even giving us half a chance for survival by announcing its presence with a symptom or two.

Doctors, themselves, believe this to be true. Thousands of gallons of blood are analyzed, millions of x-rays are taken, examinations, testing, retesting and still more testing are done and untold fortunes are spent, in part, because of the firm conviction that diseases, especially serious and fatal ones, can develop without advance warning signals (symptoms). Since both doctors and patients share this belief, all this testing seems perfectly normal.

The simple fact is that all disease creates symptoms.

A disease CANNOT exist in the body when there are no symptoms.

The reason it appears that a disease develops without any warning is that most of us, including doctors, ignore the symptoms of the early disease process. These symptoms just aren't recognized as symptoms because they don't fit into any disease category known to conventional medicine. In addition, society avoids recognizing or complaining about vague physical problems and emotional or mental symptoms. Is it any wonder that many people believe disease develops without any warning? The warnings are actually plentiful. The real problem is that they are not understood or used!

Not all the blame falls on the medical profession. Many people ignore their symptoms or do things to alter and suppress them. The result is that vital, sometimes lifesaving information is hidden or lost.

When a disease starts, the initial symptoms are usually "minor" and are generally ignored. If the person does seek medical treatment at this time, then the doctor will ignore the symptoms. All the blood analysis and other diagnostic tests will be normal and the doctor assumes he has nothing to treat.

Gradually, over time, the symptoms will get worse and more frequent. These symptoms will still generally be ignored by both the patient and the doctor. Occasionally, the patient will treat himself. The symptoms continue to get worse until a threshold is reached.

The threshold is the point at which the severity of symptoms are such that the patient is "taken seriously".

This usually occurs when a blood test is abnormal, a spot shows up on an x-ray or another physical piece of evidence has been produced by the body. It is at this moment that the patient is pronounced "ill" and requiring medical treatment. In reality, the disease process has been going on for some time.

Let's say a spot suddenly appears in the lung on a chest x-ray. It didn't just pop out full blown and big enough to be seen. That mass started as one cell, grew to 200 cells and finally reached a point (the threshold) at which it was detectable by current medical technology, the x-ray machine. The truth is that there were other noticeable symptoms including non-physical ones which the patient had before the spot showed up on the x-ray, but they were ignored. All the symptoms, both before and including the mass in the lung, are part of the same disease process. The patient was "sick" the entire time, long before the spot was visible.

The tragedy is that the current system of waiting until physical or other definite pathology is present before treating a patient is wasting the very time when the chances of complete cure are at their best. The time between the start of the disease process and when the disease has progressed to physical changes (crossing the threshold) is generally the best interval for effective, safe and permanent elimination of the disease process and its results. Treatment during this period also can completely prevent the development of the more serious and dangerous physical pathology, like the spot on the lung. Once these physical changes have occurred, the body must reverse those changes to be cured. This definitely can and frequently does occur with Homeopathic treatment, yet it can take longer than treating a disease below the threshold of destructive physical problems. Once a disease has progressed above the threshold, there are often certain irreversible changes, such as tissue destruction, that mark the point of no return and will not be reversed by any treatment. Very often a patient is incurable after the threshold has been crossed.

*Homeopathy is the ultimate preventive medicine,
curing disease before its path of destruction
has become irreversible.*

If there have been irreversible physical changes, Homeopathy can still remove the disease cause to stop further symptom development and tissue damage. Conventional medicine can be effectively used as symptomatic relief in the late stages of disease after the pathologic changes and permanent tissue damage have taken place. Then, surgery or medications can try to compensate for the permanently lost tissues and their functions. They will not cure the disease, they will only block that particular pathway of disease expression.

Historically, scientific advances and technological development have lowered the threshold level, that time when the patient is officially declared "sick" by the medical establishment. For example, advances in imaging from x-ray to CT and NMR scanners and in chemical analysis of blood have improved early detection of problems. Despite these miraculous advances, the whole focus is still limited to the physical body and the results of tests without evaluating the whole person and the limitations to personal freedom that he is experiencing.

Even with the periodic lowering of the threshold for believing a patient is really "sick", anyone still falling below the threshold continues to be disregarded and ignored. These patients are called malingerers, hypochondriacs, nuisance patients, crazy or worse. They are subjected to ridicule or contempt and referred to psychiatrists, therapists, or an endless string of other physicians. Their only fault is that they have not yet become sick enough to develop actual physical symptoms or tissue changes or they have symptoms only in the emotional or mental areas. As the threshold lowers because of growing technology, these physical and tissue changes are detected far earlier, therefore putting more of these patients into the category of the "legitimately sick".

Patients who fell below the threshold years ago and would not have been declared sick, today are seen as sick. Mitral Valve Prolapse and Chronic Fatigue - Epstein Barr Virus Syndrome are two recent examples. Does this mean that before the development of all this technology they were not just as sick as they are today? Of course not! Isn't it logical then, that patients who, today, fall below the "sick" threshold may indeed be very ill but we haven't yet developed the technology that is sensitive enough to detect the disease process? The only possible answer is yes!

There is, however, a technology already available that is sensitive enough to detect the subtle changes that occur at the very beginning of a disease. We have everything needed to move the threshold line down to the very first day of the disease! The technology is the patient. Using our comprehensive definitions of health and symptoms, any disease will present enough symptoms from its onset to alert the perceptive person of its presence. Our ability to operate and use this technology has simply been lost! It is only necessary to re-educate ourselves to observe, acknowledge and interpret all the useful and lifesaving diagnostic information that we display every moment of every day. A skilled Homeopath will do the rest.

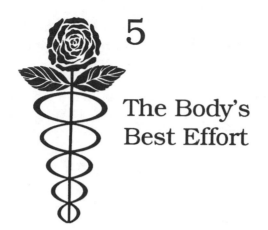

5

The Body's Best Effort

With our broader perspective on the meaning and importance of symptoms and with our expanded definitions of both health and disease, we can now examine the disease process in more detail to gain additional understanding about how Homeopathy works.

Each of us has three main areas or levels: physical, emotional and mental. These areas are separate and distinct with specific functions, characteristics and qualities, yet they are also integrated and interact in a unified way.

Symptoms can occur in all or any one of these areas. Physical symptoms are very familiar to us. They include pains, discharges, swellings or malfunctions of certain organs, resulting in a disruption of physical health.

Symptoms or disturbances in the emotional and mental functions and their contribution to disease are generally less familiar. Emotional functions include desires, feelings and affections. Mental functions include perceptions, understanding, memory and thinking abilities. A disease process that affects either of these areas will result in a disorder or improper functioning of these special attributes. All of us, at one time or another, have experienced anger, irritability, sadness, fear or excitement; these are emotional symptoms. Forgetfulness, confusion or dullness of thinking are mental symptoms. In general, any emotional or mental characteristics which limit your personal freedom are symptoms.

In biological terms, our bodies are maintained by a process known as homeostasis which is the balance, harmony, stability and equilibrium of the whole person.

Balance or homeostasis is vital to life.

All the functions of the physical, emotional and mental levels operate to maintain this balance. A change in the environment can disturb the balance and thereby begin a disease process. Your whole being reacts to the disease by trying to restore and maintain this balance.

The following example of a balance board will demonstrate what homeostasis is, how it can be disrupted by disease and how it can be restored by eliminating the disease with Homeopathic treatment.

Our balance board sits on one support. To balance it we must place equal weight on each side of the support.

Let's use the balance board to represent a person. We'll put three glasses on each side to represent the physical, emotional and mental levels. The glasses are empty meaning this person has no symptoms. The beam is perfectly balanced and in a level position, representing homeostasis. This person experiences

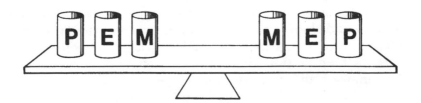

freedom: he is physically well and active, he is in harmony with his family, friends and himself, he is feeling vital, energetic and being productive.

If you were to touch the board it would rock up and down like a teeter totter and then it would gradually return to its original, balanced position. This natural resistance to distur-bance also occurs in each of us, allowing easy recovery from the small, everyday interferences that commonly happen. The healthier the person, the stronger the innate tendency is to retain a balance in spite of any disrupting influence.

A truly healthy person can be exposed to many disease-producing influences without becoming sick.

This person, like most people, has been exposed to certain adverse influences which may initiate a disease. This initiating factor could be any one of many different influences, such as: grief, emotional shock, trauma, exposure to certain kinds of weather, sleep deprivation, bad news, overwork, or mental stress to name just a few. A disease process will only start if the influence is of the right type and is strong enough to affect the person.

One such disease influence occurs and is strong enough to start a disease in this person. We'll show this by moving our balance board slightly off center.

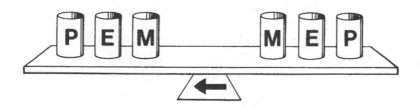

The board is now tipping to one side.

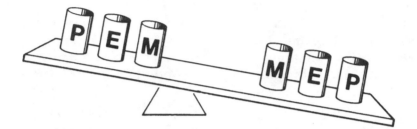

The presence of a disease has interrupted the natural balance or homeostasis in the person. If balance is not restored, the person will die. His total organism, all three levels, must respond and restore the balance any way it can. To do this, a specialized system called the Defense Mechanism has been developed. Its job is to monitor the entire person, to recognize any disturbance in the balanced state and correct it.

The most obvious way to correct the current imbalance is to move the board back to its center, the original healthy state. A strong Defense Mechanism can provide resistance to the beginning of a disease process, but it cannot remove the disease once it has started.   So it can't re-center the board now. To balance the board and make it level again in its new position, our only other choice is to add weight to the short side of the board.

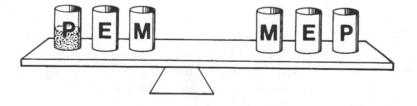

Just the right amount of sand, (symptoms in a person), not more or less, poured into the glass will restore the board to the balanced position. For the person, homeostasis is restored.

Let's say that the disturbance or disease influence which upset the homeostasis and created the imbalance was the death of this person's brother. His Defense Mechanism will create just the right amount of symptoms to compensate exactly for the disease which was started by the severe grief. In this case, it is a rash on his right forearm. The location, extent, type and intensity of the rash, or whatever symptom may be produced, are all very carefully determined by the Defense Mechanism depending on the exact requirements necessary to restore the balance or homeostasis.

Our body, through our Defense Mechanism, knows exactly what it is doing, even if we don't understand or appreciate it at the time.

This is shown in the example by the "P" or Physical glass filled with the exact amount of sand needed to restore the board to a balanced position. The balance is only made possible by the presence of the sand in the glass. The health or homeostasis of the patient also depends on the presence of the rash on his arm.

In our society we don't tolerate symptoms very well, especially visible symptoms like red, itchy rashes. This person will, undoubtedly, head straight for the doctor and ask for immediate relief. The doctor will prescribe an ointment, usually one containing cortisone. Sure enough, the rash goes away. The patient is happy, the doctor is happy, the pharmacist is happy and the drug company is happy.

Now let's see what really happened.

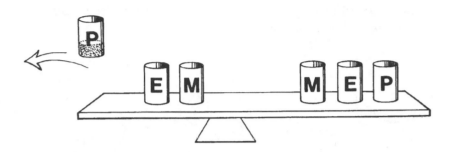

By removing the rash, or the "P" glass in our example, the board goes back the way it was before we used the sand. It is off balance again.

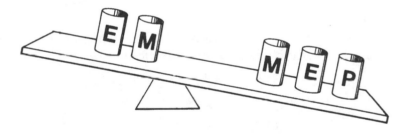

We know homeostasis or balance is a necessary condition for life. This person must now balance himself again, but without the rash. Because of the treatment, the rash is no longer available as a method for the Defense Mechanism to restore balance. Other symptoms must now be used. Physical symptoms other than the skin rash, or symptoms from other aspects of the person must be used.

We'll show this by the removal of the Physical glass. We cannot use that glass anymore to restore the balance. There are only two glasses left with which to reestablish balance, the Emotional and Mental glasses.

First, we pour sand in the "E" glass or emotional level and we move closer to our balanced position. These symptoms are irritability and sleeplessness.

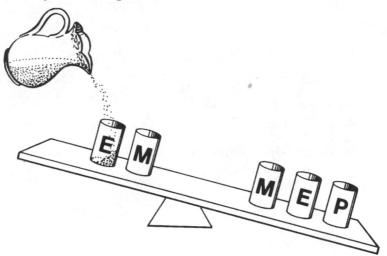

Just the right amount of sand is then added to the "M" glass, representing forgetfulness on the mental level.

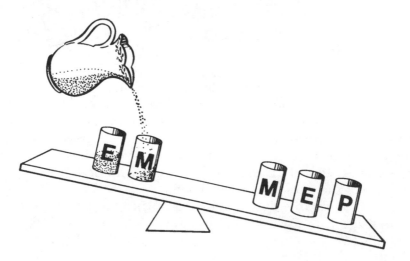

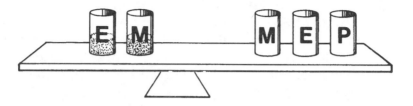

Balance is again restored by the Defense Mechanism.

It has been a year since this person's rash disappeared after using the ointment. Now he notices he is forgetting little things. He is also beginning to have arguments at work, he's irritable and having trouble sleeping at night. Off he goes to the doctor again. After all, the doctor was so successful at getting rid of his rash!

Now the patient tells the doctor: "A year ago I had a skin rash and the medicine you gave me worked wonders to get rid of it. Now, I have a different problem. I've been under a lot of stress lately. I've been a little worried because I've started to forget things. Sometimes I forget little things like where I put my keys, people's names and things like that. I haven't done anything about it because it hasn't been so bad until last week when I completely forgot a very important appointment. The client was furious and I nearly got fired. It wouldn't have been such a big deal except that I'm already in a bit of trouble at work. I've been so irritable lately that I just fly off the handle at the least little thing and I've had several big arguments. My supervisor has warned me about it and I try to control my temper, but it seems to be getting worse. I'm sure it's just the stress of the job; that and the fact that I can't sleep at night. Things just pile up on my mind and I can't turn it off. If I could just get a good night's sleep, I know I wouldn't be so irritable the next day."

Job stress seems such a logical explanation for this situation and the patient's complaints. So, the doctor will do what doctors usually do, again prescribe medications. This time he gives sleeping pills and tranquilizers. No connection is made by either the doctor or the patient between the original grief, the skin rash, its forced disappearance by the ointment and the current problems of irritability, forgetfulness and insomnia, yet they are all connected. They must be connected because a human being is only one organism with every part linked to every other part.

Nothing has been done to correct the original disease. Through all this treatment, the disease or cause of the symptoms is still present and active. It is very easy for us to see exactly what is happening using the balance board. It is much more difficult to see it in a patient, and even more difficult to see it in ourselves.

We're all under stress from time to time and we all get irritable, that's just normal, right? Wrong! Irritability is a symptom created to balance a person in a state of ill health.

We have learned to live with so much disease that we assume these problems are normal.

This is what occurred in the late 1700's in France. In one of the few medical books available at that time, the author described the normal liver as a firm organ located on the right under the ribs and extending three to six inches below the rib margin. Today we know that this describes a liver that is very sick, probably cirrhotic. In those days sanitation was very poor, making the water polluted and extremely dangerous to drink. As a result, everyone drank wine and quite a lot of it. Consequently, most people had enlarged livers. Those livers were considered normal because everybody had one. It wasn't normal, it was just common. How many symptoms, like irritability, do we accept today as *normal* just because they are so *common*?

Now, back to the patient. He is finally tired of taking all those medications and still not feeling well. He has heard about Homeopathy and decided to give it a try. Once the Homeopathic remedy is given, the disease or "cause" is eliminated. The balance board is now replaced in the center on the support. (We will discuss diagnosis and treatment in more detail in later chapters).

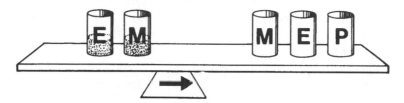

Without the disease, we expect that the board should be perfectly balanced, representing health. What we find, however, is that it is tilted again.

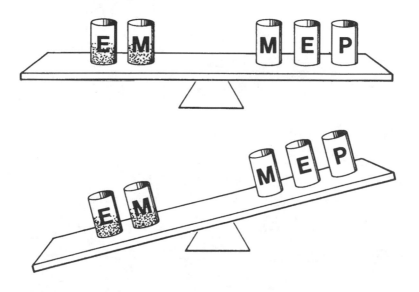

It is now the sand that is creating the imbalance instead of correcting it! The sand should be removed because it is no longer needed.

For the person, this means that after the disease or cause is removed, symptoms created earlier by the Defense Mechanism for balance and homeostasis are now interfering with proper balance. Our Defense Mechanism will then gently and safely remove all the symptoms, without additional medication, therapy, surgery or difficulty. This is the essence of true inner healing.

The first symptoms to go are the most recent ones. In this case, the sleeplessness, irritability and forgetfulness leave as shown when we remove the sand from the Emotional and Mental glasses.

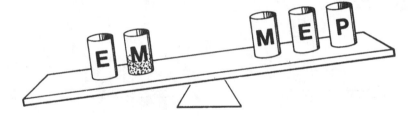

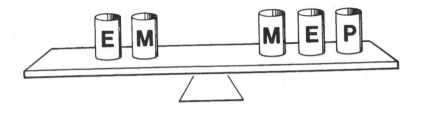

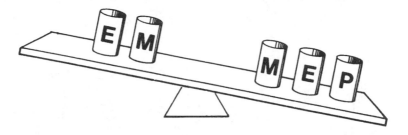

The person is still out of balance because the Physical glass is missing.

The Physical glass was removed when the cortisone was applied to get rid of the rash. The rash was not cured, it was only suppressed. This caused the other symptoms to be required. The Homeopathic remedy will cause the release of the suppressed rash, which may return in a mild form for a short time. The Physical glass, representing the rash, is repositioned on the balance board.

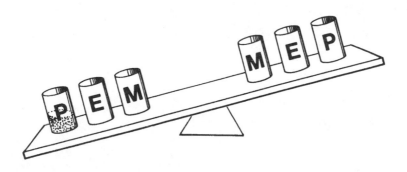

After this, the Defense Mechanism removes the rash in the same manner it removed the other symptoms. The "P" glass, too, is then emptied as the rash is removed.

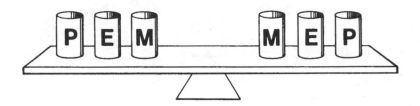

The person has returned to his normal state of good health. He is now a joyful, healthy, vital and free human being. We have witnessed a true cure.

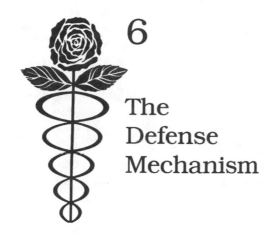

6

The
Defense
Mechanism

AHHH-CHOOOOO sniff, sniff! A little tickle in your throat, an irritating cough and that tired, achy feeling. You know that story; you're getting a cold. Why did it have to happen now, at the worst possible time, when there's so much to do? You just got over a cold, why is this happening again? What is the difference between yesterday when you felt fine and today, that caused this illness to appear?

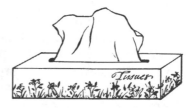

Your symptoms have developed in response to a disease process and are needed to restore balance to your body. How and why did this disease start in the first place? What happened from one day to the next to change you from a healthy person into one who now has symptoms?

You are already somewhat familiar with your system of protection, the Defense Mechanism, from our discussion of balance and homeostasis in the last chapter. The Defense

Mechanism's first duty is to prevent any influence from starting a disease process. If a disease does begin, it is the Defense Mechanism that detects the imbalance in your body and restores that balance by creating symptoms.

You are probably familiar with one aspect of the Defense Mechanism, the immune system. It functions to protect the physical body and rid it of infections and other diseases. As intricate and complex as the immune system is, the total Defense Mechanism is even more so because it protects you on all three levels: physical, emotional and mental.

The immune system with its white blood cells, lymphocytes and antibodies is much more easily understood than the Defense Mechanism because it can be seen, measured, studied, tested and evaluated. Conversely, the Defense Mechanism is more difficult to understand because it also functions on the elusive emotional and mental levels which defy direct measurement.

In recent years, the action of the Defense Mechanism on the emotional level has begun to be observed and studied. With the growing awareness and understanding of psychology, many people are aware of the psychological changes that occur in a person who has suffered through tragic events. Appropriately enough, these are called psychological "defenses" and include attitudes, reactions, thoughts, personality traits and responses. What is not generally understood is that these symptoms, like physical symptoms, are created by the Defense Mechanism to restore balance or homeostasis and are vital and necessary for a person's survival.

Just as with physical symptoms, removing or suppressing emotional symptoms can often result in the development of more serious symptoms. I am not suggesting that they should be left alone or ignored. Quite the contrary; they do require treatment. The disease process that required their presence must be properly treated and removed. These emotional symptoms will then be naturally corrected and cured by the same mechanisms that created them in the first place.

Your Defense Mechanism operates continually to protect you from ever-present disease influences. We often think that we stay healthy because we avoid stress, germs or other disease producing factors. This is certainly not so. We are constantly being confronted with potential disease as we live and work in this stressful, germ laden world. These stresses and other disease causing factors are always present.

There are two factors that work together to determine whether you will stay healthy or become ill, and both are equally important. The first factor is the strength and functioning of your Defense Mechanism and the second is the strength of the disease influence or cause.

There is an intricate dance between these two factors, Defense and Disease, each playing a vital role.

When a disease influence confronts us and our Defense Mechanism, there are four possible outcomes. In the first possibility, our Defense Mechanism is so much stronger than any incoming disease force that we are not even aware that it is protecting us! Potential disease influences are simply repelled or "brushed aside" seemingly without effort as the Defense Mechanism works "invisibly" in our favor. We just go about our life, doing what we want with health, vitality, energy, creativity and happiness. We are completely unaware of the resistance we have which keeps us from getting sick at any given moment.

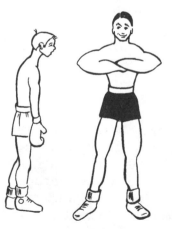

In the second of our four possibilities, the disease is much stronger than the Defense Mechanism. Overwhelmed by the disease, the Defense Mechanism does not have the ability to create the needed symptoms to restore balance. There may not even be enough symptoms possible to enable the balance to be maintained. Without homeostasis or balance, the result is death.

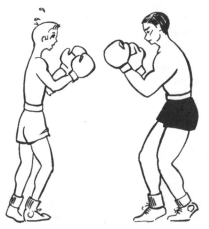

In the third possibility, the Defense Mechanism is confronted by a disease which has enough power to cause a disturbance but which is still not as strong as the Defense Mechanism. The Defense Mechanism then activates the appropriate physical, emotional and mental symptoms to combat and counteract the disease influence.

All your symptoms are tangible pieces of evidence that your Defense Mechanism is "battling it out" with the disease process. When the Defense Mechanism finally has the strength to overpower the disease, the battle is over. The symptoms that were necessary to combat the disease are eliminated; harmony and health are re-established. This is known as an acute, or self-limiting disease. We are all familiar with these illnesses. The symptoms may last for several days or even a couple of weeks. When they finally resolve, our normal state of health is restored. Most of us don't realize that this is the proper performance of our Defense Mechanism; creating the symptoms (about which we usually complain bitterly) and effecting the cure so health returns.

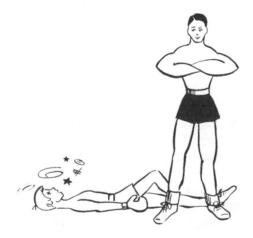

The fourth and final possibility is by far the most common. The disease influence is, again, strong enough to interfere and initiate a disease causing the Defense Mechanism to produce symptoms. Neither side is quite strong enough to overpower the other. The result is a chronic, long term "fight" between the Defense Mechanism and the disease process.

Since the disease is never completely eliminated, symptoms will continually be required to compensate for its activity.

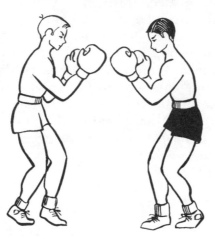

This process can last for months, years or even a lifetime. All chronic diseases, persistent symptoms or conditions for which a person must take daily medications, are a result of this process.

We have seen that the Defense Mechanism has the enormous job of keeping us healthy on a daily basis. Continuous small changes are constantly being made to adjust to the ever shifting and sometimes volatile nature of life and living.

A good example of how the Defense Mechanism maintains equilibrium is a modern, climate controlled high-rise office building.

In the building there are many factors that must be kept constant, such as the temperature, humidity and oxygen content of the air. Other factors such as lighting and security locks on the doors will vary with the time of day, but these too

will change on a regulated schedule. There is a central processing station that monitors these and other parameters within the
building.

When the temperature out-
side falls, more heat will be generated inside the building. If the
outside climate gets hotter, then
the air conditioning comes on to
bring the room temperature back
within the comfort range. At night,
after everyone has gone home,
certain lights will turn off and
others will still be required. Any
disturbance or change in the environment will be detected and
the appropriate compensation will
be made. The central processing
station functions continuously to
ensure a constant environment,
maintaining all the parameters
within their preset range.

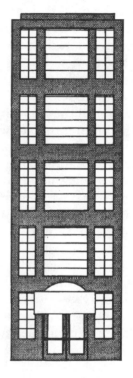

When there is a change in
temperature or some other parameter, the cause is not generally known. If the temperature
drops, it may be due to the
weather outside or to a large in-
crease in the number of people going in and out of the building
and opening the doors. The central processing station makes
the necessary adjustment even though the cause of the change
is not directly known. All that is needed is to detect the change
itself. As long as the changes are within the range that the
central processing station is designed to handle, the proper
adjustments can always be made.

The people in the building conduct their business in
comfort without even a thought about all this. The properly

functioning system is designed to be "invisible". It is so automatic that no attention needs to be directed to the office environment at all. Only if the system stops functioning, the lights go out after dark or the temperature becomes too hot or too cold would they even be aware of it.

This is exactly how the Defense Mechanism functions. There are certain parameters, in fact millions of them, that must be kept within specific ranges to maintain homeostasis or balance. Each parameter has a normal and healthy range that is unique to it.

Some of these parameters, such a body temperature, sleep and available sugar or water, are very familiar to us. Thousands of others, vital to our proper functioning, are less well known. Enzymes which carry out chemical processes must be kept at certain levels, blood flow must be regulated to ensure that its distribution is appropriate for both immediate and long term needs of various organs and other cells, alterations in nerve activity are required to regulate muscles and other organ functions. Hormones, nutrients, chemical mediators, mental and emotional activities, oxygen, fluid balance and thousands of other parameters are constantly adjusted in response to a dynamic environment. It is a huge job for the Defense Mechanism always to maintain balance.

Just as in our example of the modern high-rise building, as long as the kinds and extent of the adjustments needed are within the range of the Defense Mechanism, our body will function properly and health will be maintained. We will be totally unaware of the great amount of automatic activity that is going on at every single moment.

Why did your symptoms develop when they did? The answer is simple. At that exact moment, the disease influence, whatever it was, was just enough stronger than your Defense Mechanism that symptoms were produced to re-establish a balanced state. The result is the disease and its effect: ACHOO, sniff, sniff!

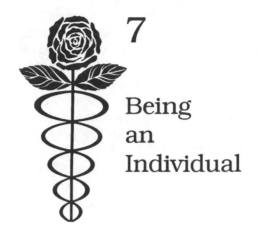

7

Being an Individual

Jane and Hank went to their favorite restaurant and had dinner. Both ordered the same dish. That night, Hank had a terrible stomach ache that kept him awake all night. Jane slept just fine and had no ill effects after the meal.

Sarah and Dylan were out in the yard raking the leaves on a cold and crisp Autumn day. Their efforts were often foiled by the blustery wind. That night, Sarah had a terrible ear ache and a fever. Dylan slept just fine. The effects of the yard work on him were only evident the next day when he woke up with a sore, stiff and painful back.

Why do different people develop different sets of symptoms when exposed to the same kind of disease influ-

ence? What explanation is there for the great variety of ways
that each person will express a disease process?

The set of symptoms that our Defense Mechanism creates
in response to a disease can vary and is specific to each of us.
How does that happen? How does your Defense Mechanism
decide what symptoms to produce for you?

To explain this, I'll use something familiar, a pair of jeans.
We all wear them, so we all know where they wear out. The leg
ends get frayed, the knees wear out, and the pockets get holes
where the wallet is kept. Often, the belt loops come off.

Jeans develop a particular kind of wear and tear from the
stresses they encounter. They become "diseased" in very
characteristic ways, determined both by the stresses and their
particular kind of fabric and style.

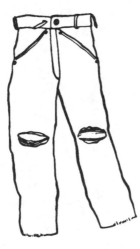 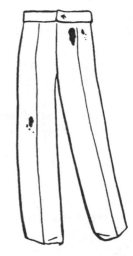

Now let's consider another pair of pants, dress slacks. They are made of silk and used for more formal occasions. In many ways they resemble jeans: both have two legs, hems and a waist band. The wear and tear for dress pants is much different from jeans. There are no pockets to wear out. The seams on the sides might pull loose because the fabric isn't very strong. They will stain easily. The zipper could break or the hook at the top of the zipper may become loose or fall off. We can see that these pants, too, have a very characteristic type of wear determined by their fabric, style and the stresses particular to them.

Although the jeans and dress slacks are both pants, they have differing patterns of wear and tear. These differences result from the various stresses to which they are subjected, their fabric, style and use.

Your constitution is your inherent structure and your innate qualities, in other words, it is your very "fabric". These qualities influence and determine who you are, how you are and what you enjoy doing in your life. Your constitution is also important in determining how strong a disease force is required to start a disease process, your natural resistance to disease and what kinds of symptoms you will get if a disease does start. It also determines the kinds of stresses to which you are particularly susceptible.

Your nature and constitution determine your reactions to stresses.

This is, in part, the reason Homeopathy pays so much attention to individual reactions and symptoms. Symptoms are determined more by our susceptibilities, vulnerabilities and constitution than by the specific provoking factor or stress.

Imagine what would happen if someone stepped on the tail of every animal in the zoo. The lion would roar, the cow would moo, the cat would meow, the mouse would squeak, the sheep would bleet and the snake would hiss. The provoking event or stressor is exactly the same. The difference in the sounds produced by the animals depends on their individual constitutions.

We too respond to stresses and disease influences in our own unique way.

The stressor or disease influence is important because it begins the disease process and necessitates the symptoms. It is generally not as important in determining the specific kind of symptoms you will develop. This is influenced by your individual constitution and your Defense Mechanism.

To demonstrate the idea of constitutional susceptibility further, let's look at an automobile tire. During manufacture, a defect develops which leaves one area thinner than the rest of the tire. This is an inherent quality of the tire, part of its "constitution". Under normal conditions and without stresses, we don't notice this weakened area.

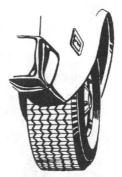

Let's see what happens when a stress or "cause" occurs. If we increase the air pressure, a bulge developes because the weakened area is not strong enough maintain the tire's shape. The exact location, size, shape and extent of the bulge and how much extra pressure is required to produce it are determined by the particular qualities or "constitution" of that tire. A minor thinning of the wall would hold up fairly well, but a significant thinning would not tolerate much increase in pressure.

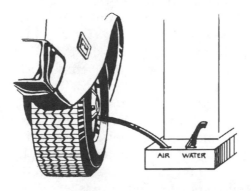

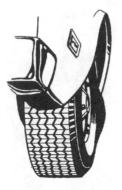

The bulge started because of the increased air pressure. It was a stress to which the thin wall was particularly susceptible. Other kinds of tire stresses such as rainy weather, bad road conditions, or heat would not affect the tire's weak point. Only under the stress of the extra pressure (cause), does the weakened area show (constitution).

This is exactly how it is with human beings. We all have these specific "weak points" where the disease will present itself if we become stressed in a certain way. Information about your weak points and the kinds of stresses which most affect you is vital to the Homeopath in making an accurate assessment of your overall condition and in choosing the correct Homeopathic remedy for you. The Homeopathic remedy improves your constitution. It "patches up" the weak spots, so you will no longer be vulnerable in those areas. You will then be more resistant to the stresses that usually affect you and less likely to produce those symptoms.

The constitution is only one of several important factors determining why people react differently to stress and disease influences. We still need to explain how the Defense Mechanism chooses specific symptoms to restore a healthy balance. To do this we need to look more closely at our three main areas of functioning: physical, emotional and mental.

We are generally most familiar with the physical level. The emotional and mental aspects are recognized, but their role in disease and symptom development is less well appreciated. We can best understand these three levels and their interactions by first describing the physical level and then demonstrating how the principles and ideas shown there also apply in each of the other levels.

Within the physical level, there are many different organs and types of tissues. Each organ system performs very specialized functions. It is shaped and designed to best suit the specific job it is expected to do. For example, one function of the lungs is the collection of oxygen from the air for absorption into the blood stream. The shape, location, cellular components and chemical composition of the lungs are specifically designed to accomplish this as well as other goals.

Everywhere in the physical body,
both structure and function are
inextricably linked together.
Form follows function.

By examining one specific lung function, oxygen absorption, we can learn more about how the body functions in health and disease states. The lungs control how much or how little oxygen absorbtion takes place by altering how many times you breathe each minute. This respiratory rate can range from slow to rapid. Any of these rates could be normal or a sign of disease depending on the situation and your overall condition. An accelerated rate is normal when you exercise and a low rate is normal during sleep. On the other hand, an accelerated rate is a symptom of disease if someone is hyperventilating after a shock and a low respiratory rate can be a symptom when it results from a head injury.

A slow or rapid respiratory rate, by itself, does not determine whether it is a symptom. Its significance can only be determined by evaluating it in the terms of the whole person.

The functions of the other organ systems, such as the gastro-intestinal, circulatory, musculo-skeletal and neuological systems, operate in a similar manner. Each has a specific function with a range of possible action. Many symptoms are normal activities that occur at an inappropriate time or under inappropriate circumstances. Now let's apply this idea to the emotional and mental areas and their symptoms.

The emotional level with its variety of emotions can be thought of in the same way as the physical body with its different organ systems. Like all physical organ systems, each human emotion has specific purposes, characteristics, functions and a wide range of action. The temperament, character, desires and preferences are a few of the "organ systems" in the emotional realm. Specific functions are the individual emotions such as anger, irritability, joy, jealousy, excitement, sadness, timidity and grief. Many of us may regard some of these emotions as "negative" or undesirable. In fact, there are many different therapy techniques designed to eliminate these "bad" emotions.

Each emotion
has a very important function and
is necessary for our health.

Emotions are generally not thought of as specialized functions similar to the physical organ systems. Since there are no conventional names for these functional areas on the emotional level, we'll create our own. There is a system of the emotion level which functions to protect us in stressful situations. We'll call it "reaction one".

"Reaction one" protects us by responding to stress with the emotions it generates. It too, like the lung, has a wide range of possible actions for doing this. On one end of the range is anger and on the other end is indifference. It also can produce many emotions between these two.

All the emotions in this system are useful and necessary for our survival. Just as we saw in the description of the lung and the respiratory rate, each of these emotions can be a healthy or an unhealthy response depending on the situation. Typically, anger is regarded as a "negative" emotion. There are many times, when being angry is appropriate, and therefore, is a healthy response. It can even be potentially life saving. Anger is a reasonable and appropriate reaction if, for example, someone purposely lies to you or you are unjustly fired from your job. On the other end of the scale is indifference. This emotion, like anger, is also generally thought of as undesirable. It too can be an appropriate and healthy response, allowing you to be detached in specific situations.

Both anger and indifference also can be symptoms. For example, indifference to your family, friends or even your own life are symptoms requiring treatment. Anger over insignificant events or on a constant and chronic basis show this emotion as a symptom. Whether it is a normal, healthy response or a symptom depends on the events around the experience of the emotion. Using our comprehensive definition of health assists in deciding whether a characteristic or emotional state is a sign of disease or not. If the overall freedom of the person is limited by the emotion, then it is a symptom.

These principles also apply to our mental level. The mind has specific areas of function such as memory, understanding, thought, problem solving and ideas. Examples of symptoms on the mental level are forgetfulness, confusion, slowness of thinking, psychosis and even schizophrenia.

The different levels can each produce symptoms which reflect the functions that normally operate there. Trauma to the physical body can result in pain, bleeding, swelling or drainage. Trauma to the emotions, such as a disappointment or grief also results in pain, but it is exhibited in an entirely different way. Pain in the emotions can be expressed as weeping, insomnia, sadness or apathy. The response to trauma on the mental level is different still, with the symptoms including difficulty concentrating, forgetfulness or inability to think clearly.

All three levels are interconnected and when presented with a disease process, will respond in a unified way. The Defense Mechanism will do whatever is necessary to maintain homeostasis or balance. It chooses symptoms in a very precise and carefully calculated manner, creating just enough symptoms, and no more. It creates the most minor or innocuous symptom it can in the least vital area of the organism. If more symptoms are needed, then and only then, will a slightly more important structure or system be involved in producing the symptoms.

The Defense Mechanism uses a hierarchy of symptoms to determine what symptoms will be created and when, always protecting the most vital structures and functions. They are always the last to be involved.

This hierarchy is similar in principle to the functioning of the city-states during the Middle Ages.

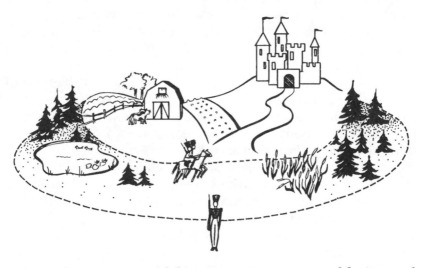

On the perimeter of the city-state, a group of foot guards patrols the borders. They are protecting the fields and forests of the outlying countryside. They are ready to fight off any invaders. A single invader trying to get by this circle of guards wouldn't get very far. Should a larger army attack, the border guards would be over run and the city-state would loose its first line of defense. The land that the foot guards protected would also be lost. While unfortunate, this would not severely impact the city-state as a whole.

The next barrier against invasion is the mounted soldiers. The soldiers are very important because they are the last line of defense protecting the fields where the food grows. If these mounted soldiers fall, the city-state would suffer serious hardship from the loss of that farming land. Since the border guards were overrun by the enemy, the mounted guards are called into action. An even stronger defense is maintained near the castle in the center.

The total amount of defense is limited, so it must be used in a very logical and efficient way. There is a hierarchy of community resources that require protection. Forests, fields, water, food, farmland, citizens, treasury and the King are all protected, according to their value to the country and the soldiers are stationed accordingly. Each level of defense protects a more vital part of the community's resources. The King is behind the strongest defense of all.

Our own hierarchy and Defense System is organized in a very similar way, it protects the most vital structures with the greatest defense. We know that when a disease process starts, the Defense Mechanism will create just the right set of symptoms to compensate and counteract the disease process. The Defense Mechanism knows exactly which symptoms are needed, and at what intensity. It follows the hierarchical order exactly.

To understand this process more fully, let's create a simple hierarchy. Looking at just the physical level: a small patch of rash on the skin is not nearly as concerning as a throbbing pain in a joint. The pain in the joint is not as significant as a pain in the heart. Already we can see an order of importance in the organs themselves. What if the rash covered half your body? Then it would be of far greater concern than a single joint pain. It might even represent a greater danger to life than a minor pain in your heart. In addition to the location and type of symptom, the intensity or severity is an important consideration in symptom placement on the hierarchical scale.

Naturally, the hierarchy also must include our emotional and mental areas. In general, the mind and its functions are the most vital to us. It is our ability to think, reason and have free will that makes us unique and truly human. Therefore our mind is the most highly guarded. Typically, after the mind, the emotions are most guarded and finally the physical body. These levels are not in a distinct, clear cut, linear hierarchy. There is an intricate interplay of all three levels that results in the final hierarchy used by the Defense Mechanism. George Vithoulkas, a master Homeopath, writes extensively about this concept in his book *The Science of Homeopathy*.

Let's explore our hierarchy further. Which of these symptoms is preferable: persistent episodes of sneezing or a stomach ulcer? Irritability or lung cancer? Hives or panic attacks? With these obvious examples, it is easy to see the hierarchical order of symptoms. In the first example, we are comparing two physical symptoms while in the last two examples we are contrasting symptoms from both the emotional level and the physical body. Irritability has a far less serious impact on us than lung cancer and hives have a far less limiting effect than panic attacks. In one situation, the physical symptom is more serious than the emotional; in the other, the reverse is true. The placement of these symptoms in the hierarchical order is not determined solely by the physical, emotional or mental levels from which they come. It is determined, instead, by the limitation of freedom which the symptom imposes on our total functioning as a human being.

It is widely thought that both the emotions and the mind cause physical problems. The simultaneous appearance of a specific emotion or a way of thinking and a physical symptom has lead many people to connect the two. All, however, are symptoms created by the Defense Mechanism in response to the presence of a disease process. It is disease which causes the physical, emotional and mental symptoms, they do not cause each other. This is a subtle yet very important distinction.

This hierarchy is a very complex system of organizing all

possible symptoms and their varying intensities. Your heredity, constitution and vitality all influence this order.   The
Defense Mechanism follows this order in a very precise and
exacting way.

When any symptom appears, there are several things you
can rely on as biological fact. The first is that a disease process
has started and your body is responding through its Defense
Mechanism in a very appropriate and necessary way to maintain homeostasis or balance. The second fact is that the precise
symptom selected is the very lowest on your hierarchical scale
and therefore the least limiting to your healthy freedom.
Finally, and most importantly, in the presence of a disease
process, your mind, emotions and body, work together to
maintain the best possible state of health for you at all times.

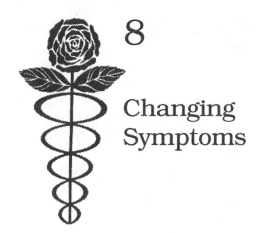

8

Changing Symptoms

All possible symptoms are placed in hierarchical order and the Defense Mechanism then chooses which symptoms to use at any given time in its efforts to combat disease. All symptoms in a person are related to each other because they are all manifestations of the same disease process. No symptom can possibly be considered an isolated event, independent of the functioning and health of the whole person. As a unified, integrated living organism, each of us can only express disease in this unified way.

Symptoms can change as the disease changes by increasing in severity or improving through healing. Sometimes these transformations involve different organ systems or functions. We illustrated this in chapter five with the example of the balance beam. In response to the disease process, the Defense Mechanism first created a skin rash and when the same disease later deepened, it then developed forgetfulness, insomnia and irritability.

The idea that one disease can produce a variety of symptoms that can change from one to another is new to most people.

In fact, it is also new to most doctors.

This basic idea, that an underlying state can be expressed in a variety of forms, is not a new concept in nature. The rainbow or light spectrum illustrates this idea. On one end is the color red, and on the other is purple. Orange, yellow, green, blue, and violet are in between and are shown in a continuous array of color. All the colors are made from light, and each is made by a different wave length and frequency.

The wave length is the actual length of one single wave of light. The frequency is the number of light waves over a given amount of time. The color red is produced by a very long wave length that has a low frequency. On the other end of the spectrum, purple is produced by a very short wave length with a high frequency. All the other colors are produced by varying these two factors between the values for red and those for purple. On a light spectrum, it is possible to go from one color to another simply by changing the wave length. The underlying condition, light, does not change.

As another example, let's look at what happens to water at different temperatures. Water can either be steam, liquid or ice simply by altering its temperature. Thus, water is changing its form, going up and down the "consistency scale", by changing its temperature.

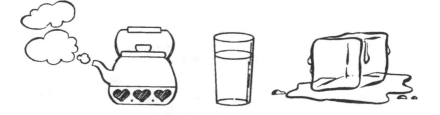

In a similar way, symptoms too can change. Your symptoms all arise from one disease process just as all colors come from light and there are several different forms of water. For light, the changing factor is wave length. For water, the determining factor is temperature. For symptoms, the distinguishing factor is the extent and severity of the disease process.

You travel up and down
your hierarchy of symptoms
reflecting a change in your health.

As the disease process becomes more severe, our bodies require symptoms of a more extensive nature to counteract the increasing strength of the disease. The less serious symptoms go away and are replaced by more serious ones that can serve the purpose of restoring the appropriate balance.

Taking this idea one step further, we can draw a chart of symptoms similar to the continuous spectrum of light. On one end are the symptoms used when the disease process is minimal and on the other end are the symptoms occurring when the disease process is severe. The symptoms change depending on the level or severity of the disease process.

Thus, hayfever can turn into asthma as the disease process progresses. A skin rash can turn into depression, arthritis can turn into heart disease, an ear infection can turn into irritability. Frequently, these individual symptoms are regarded as separate diseases. For example, an asthmatic child is said to "out grow" his asthma. In fact, he is "growing into" a more serious symptom presentation of the same disease process. Because this change in level of the hierarchy may take years to develop, problems which occur later are usually regarded as new and separate diseases. All of these problems, however, are connected. All are different symptoms of the same disease process.

A few years ago, while visiting the island of Maui, I observed a good example for this concept of changing symptoms. My friends and I decided to drive to the top of Haleakala, the highest volcano on the island. Our journey started at the beach where it was extremely warm, sunny and clear. There the palm trees, bougainvillea, hibiscus, bird of paradise and other tropical plants flourished. Further inland, it got even hotter. As we began our ascent to the volcano, I noticed the tropical plants were disappearing and being replaced by other kinds of plants. In the foothills of the mountains, the temperature began to cool somewhat. Soon, we came to a Eucalyptus forest and even further up the gently inclining mountainside, there was a pine forest. The temperature was now noticeably cooler. Here I saw plants and shrubs that grow in my home state of Washington with its rainy and chilly weather. As we continued to climb, the temperature dropped even more. The trees disappeared leaving only small shrubs and plants in their place. At the top of the volcano, there was no vegetation at all. The wind was howling and cold and there was snow on the ground!

There is a very dramatic change in foliage along this "scale" extending from the shore line to the mountain top. As the climate, temperature, oxygen content and moisture changed along the "scale", determined by elevation, the kind of vegetation also changed dramatically. Each plant or tree has a set of conditions in which it grows best. When the exact amount of heat, rainfall, sunlight and other factors that suit a specific plant are present, then that plant will flourish. It cannot grow in any other environment. The pine trees cannot grow in the intense heat of the lowland planes, just as the hibiscus will not grow in the chilly altitudes of the mountain side. Each has a very precise set of requirements for its survival and optimum growth. Symptoms work the same way.

*Each symptom has
very definite requirements
for its development.*

When the conditions of disease activity, position on the hierarchy and strength of the Defense Mechanism are exactly what is required, then a specific symptom will develop. It will remain until any one of these conditions changes. It is possible to change the nature of the symptoms by altering these conditions just as the vegetation in Maui changed when the elevation and the growing conditions changed.

Let's expand this idea by drawing a scale similar to that of the mountainside. Here we will use conditions relevant to symptom development rather than changes in elevation. The main factors determining the presence of disease and the kind, intensity and severity of symptoms are the strength of the Defense Mechanism, the strength of the Disease and the interaction between them. These two factors, the Disease and the Defense Mechanism are inversely related to each other; the stronger the defense , the weaker the disease. As the defense decreases in strength, the disease increases in strength. I've arbitrarily selected the numbers on the scale just to explain these ideas. We will frequently refer to these graphs in later chapters.

Along the left side, the scale signifies the amount of activity of the Defense Mechanism. The 100% marked at the top, represents full activity. At this level, no disease can be present and there is perfect health. The stronger the Defense Mechanism, shown by being nearer to the top of the chart, the less likely a disease influence will affect us.

Moving down the scale, the decreasing numbers show a decline in function of the Defense Mechanism. Simultaneously, the disease is increasing in strength.

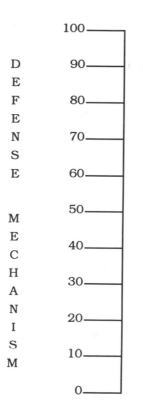

There are different symptoms present at each level on the graph. Their position is determined by the hierarchical order set by the Defense Mechanism. This graph shows how symptoms change from one to the other as the defense and disease conditions change.

This scale is similar to the light spectrum discussed earlier. It is possible to change the color of the light by changing the wave length. In this scale, the symptoms change as the amount of defense changes, from a strong Defense Mechanism at the top, to a very weakened one at the bottom.

A disease influence must be even stronger than our Defense Mechanism to overcome that defense and have an impact on us. Ordinary disease influences will not have an impact when we have a fully functional, healthy Defense Mechanism. The events that can initiate a weakening of the Defense Mechanism include emotional events such as grief, shock, excitement, weather conditions, mental strain, fear, humiliation, overwork, lack of sleep or worry.

Any weakening of the defense allows the disease to strengthen, moving the person further down the scale to a different symptom. A strong Defense Mechanism keeps the disease as limited as possible so only minor symptoms need to be developed. Each new stage of the disease process requires new or intensified symptoms. The position on the scale will reflect this change.

As the progression of the disease overcomes the Defense Mechanism, a more vital part of us developes symptoms. Again, the hierarchical order determines which symptoms interfere least with our total functioning. We saw this in the city-state when it was attacked. As the defense barriers were overcome, the enemy (or disease) progressed further and further into more vital portions of the country.

In this example, the strength of the disease influence is just enough to overcome the Defense Mechanism and cause a reduction to a function of 95%. A state of imbalance now exists. The Defense Mechanism will develop symptoms to restore the balance. (See the graph on the next page.)

At this level, the person is still very healthy. The Defense Mechanism is operating at a 95% rate and the symptoms will be quite mild. For example, the symptoms could be a runny nose, sneezing, mild headaches, irritability, the "common cold", "flu" or minor skin problems. Because these are generally regarded as benign at best and a nuisance at worst, they are usually ignored or treated with nonprescription medications aimed at symptomatic relief. Nothing has been done to cure the disease cause or to improve the functioning of the Defense Mechanism.

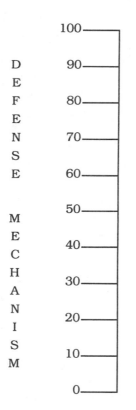

The Defense Mechanism can not overcome the disease process, so a chronic condition begins. The original symptoms will still go away, but good health will not be restored. The person will never quite feel well again after the initial problem or the old symptoms return at frequent intervals. Symptomatic relief was just that, removal of a symptom or two without improving the Defense Mechanism which is still functioning at a level of 95%. After the first symptoms have disappeared, the continued presence of the disease influence will cause new symptoms to appear.

Sometimes, the Defense Mechanism is able to overcome the disease force by itself and return to optimum functioning at 100%. Typically, however, some treatment must be given to restore the Defense Mechanism. Once it returns to the 100 % level, the "cold" or "flu" disappears. These symptoms can't exist when the Defense Mechanism is fully functional.

This is true even when bacteria are present. Germs, bacteria or viruses can only live in us if we have a reduced Defense Mechanism. When the deficiency in the Defense Mechanism is corrected and it is strong again, it has the capacity to eliminate bacteria and other germs.

Homeopathy acts by increasing the function of your Defense Mechanism , so it can overcome the disease entirely.

Unfortunately, the person being discussed isn't aware of Homeopathy so they either ignore or treat their own symptoms with medication for symptomatic relief. The initial cause of the Defense Mechanism's decline was not treated; only its effects, the specific symptoms, received any attention. The disappearance of the symptoms through this kind of treatment often occurs because the Defense Mechanism continues to deteriorate. This lower level requires different symptoms to counteract the stronger disease process.

Since the Defense Mechanism uses symptoms to signal that there is an active disease, it is difficult if not impossible for the person to be aware of the continued presence of the disease until new symptoms appear.

The person has ignored his current symptoms. When the Defense Mechanism is functioning at 95%, his symptoms are so minor that ignoring them doesn't seem to cause any problems. Typically, they go away by themselves, and that is why most people tend to ignore them.

The Defense Mechanism's efficiency will now drop to 90%.

This drop is actually the real reason that the initial symptoms went away! Symptoms which develop at a level of 95%, cannot develop at 90%. It is this disappearance of symptoms in response to the decreased efficiency of the Defense Mechanism that often convinces both the patient and his doctor that he is cured of his problems.

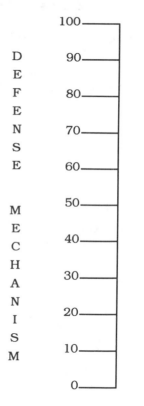

100——   HEALTH

                        SNEEZING

D   90——   **SORE THROAT, COUGH**
E
F   80——
E
N   70——
S
E   60——

M   50——
E
C   40——
H
A   30——
N
I   20——
S
M   10——

          0——

The continued deterioration of the Defense Mechanism allows a further progression of the disease process. There is now a need for increased intensity and variety of symptoms to compensate for the deepening disease. These symptoms can come from any aspect of the person including the emotional or mental areas. For most people, including conventional medical doctors, the presence of symptoms in a different part of the body or in the mind or emotions is not considered part of the previous illness, each symptom or set of related symptoms being regarded as an entirely separate disease. The current trend toward medical specialists and subspecialists compounds this problem, as few look at the patient as a whole person. Specialists are mainly concerned with the effects of a disease on the segment of the body in which they specialize.

The Defense Mechanism requires more and more symptoms to react to the ever increasing disease process. The new symptoms still follow the hierarchy of the least limiting symptoms possible that can meet the disease force and restore the balance.

Because the defense activity is now reduced to 90%, the patient has new symptoms and different intensities of the previous symptoms. The original runny nose and sneezing has now disappeared and a sore throat, cough, sleeplessness and fatigue have taken its place. These sound like symptoms of the "common cold". What we call a "cold" is typically many different kinds of symptoms associated with a slight reduction in our Defense Mechanism. I'm still waiting for the day when a patient comes to my office complaining of a decline in his Defense Mechanism instead of a cold!

The progressive decline of the Defense Mechanism allows the extension of the disease process and an increase in symptoms. It is likely that a viral growth in the nose, throat or sinuses has also occurred. This person is now so uncomfortable that he goes to the doctor for treatment, which usually includes antibiotics. Doctors know that antibiotics do not affect viruses, only bacteria. It has always amazed me how many antibiotics are prescribed for conditions like this one where no bacteria are present at all. When the patient demands "something" to help him, the hurried doctor frequently finds it easier to meet the patient's expectations with a prescription than to explain that the antibiotics will not affect the viruses.

By the way, both doctor and patient are convinced these viruses are causing the symptoms.

Here again, the treatment is only symptomatic and does nothing to improve and restore the full functioning of the Defense Mechanism. The administration of antibiotics or any other medications, if they have any affect at all, will serve to further disguise the symptoms the Defense Mechanism is producing.

The patient, having "gotten over" this episode, is unaware of the state of his Defense Mechanism. Eventually another set of symptoms will appear as a result of further decline in the defense function. This may not occur right away, in fact it usually doesn't happen immediately.

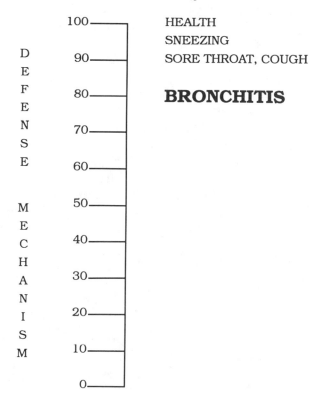

Now the Defense Mechanism has dropped to 80% efficiency and the patient is getting bronchitis several times a year. The rattling cough, fever, chest pain and fatigue are treated each time with antibiotics, cough syrup, antihistamines and aspirin. The patient also has a change in temperament; he is more irritable, easily angered and is having difficulty remembering things. So noticeable and limiting are these kinds of repeated illnesses, that both the patient and the doctor are well aware that something is wrong. Often the problem is called "lowered resistance", but there is nothing in the typical doctor's little black bag to correct that.

As the Defense Mechanism declines even further, the bronchitis episodes will go away too. Again, this is because the amount of defense has dropped to a level below that requiring the development of bronchitis. The patient is very relieved to be out of this horrible stage in his life! The doctor is convinced that the antibiotics and other medications finally worked to cure the patient.

It may be quite a while, months or even years, before the results of the patient's true state of ill health become known. The patient has now dropped to a level of 65% where pneumonia is a likely occurrence. Pneumonia cannot develop when the Defense Mechanism has a strength and functioning greater than 65%. Now the effects of many months or years of continued deterioration of the Defense Mechanism results in such a low level of function that symptoms as strong and as serious as pneumonia are required to maintain balance.

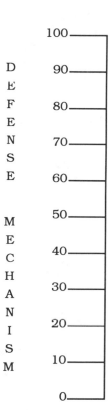

DEFENSE

100 ──── HEALTH
         SNEEZING
 90 ──── SORE THROAT, COUGH

 80 ──── BRONCHITIS

 70 ────

 PNEUMONIA

 60 ────

MECHANISM

 50 ────

 40 ────

 30 ────

 20 ────

 10 ────

  0 ────

A further drop to 55% may result in severe asthma, a chronic condition. The patient will no longer have pneumonia, bronchitis, or any of the previous conditions.

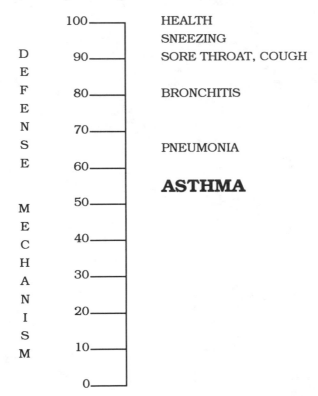

At this level, the patient will not get "colds" or other minor acute illnesses, he is far too ill. The Defense Mechanism is too depleted to produce those symptoms that are located on a higher level of the graph. This is generally the reason that people with serious or chronic conditions often say "I'm healthy except for the arthritis" or "Except for my heart condition, I'm the picture of health." To them, health means not getting acute illnesses like colds. I get nervous when someone says that they never get a cold. I wonder what they *are* getting!

Let's remember the example of the city-state being invaded. The presence of its active defense resisting the advancing enemy produced a battle. If the country had no defense at all, then the enemy would have taken over without a fight.

Symptoms are the fight.

In the human being, it is the presence of a healthy, functioning Defense Mechanism resisting advancing disease that is responsible for developing symptoms. A certain level of health is required to even produce symptoms. Contrary to conventional thought, the absence of specific symptoms frequently means a compromised state of health.

At each level of the Defense Mechanism specific kinds of symptoms will appear. In this person, all the symptoms were related to the respiratory tract. This can and does happen frequently. As we have discovered, with an active disease, symptoms can show up in any area or level that is the highest on the hierarchy and is appropriate for the severity of the disease process. Here are two more of the many possibilities involving different organ systems. (See the graph on the next page.)

These "pathways" are distinct for each of us, yet they still follow predictable patterns.

Let's look a little deeper into the differences between conventional medicine and Homeopathy. Conventional physicians don't understand that one mechanism creates all these different symptoms. Their misunderstanding is evident because they are taught to believe these individual symptoms are different diseases. Conventional medicine has made observations that certain kinds of symptoms tend to be related. They know that many people with asthma also have skin problems, that arthritis often follows a long history of psoriasis. Unfortunately, the conventional medical world has not carried this to

100	HEALTH	HEALTH
	SKIN RASH	RUNNY NOSE
90	IRRITABILITY	NASAL CONGESTION
		EAR INFECTIONS
80	INDIGESTION	HAYFEVER
	SUGAR CRAVING	SHYNESS
70	ANGER	FEAR OF AIRPLANES
	JOINT PAIN	DESIRES SALTY FOODS
60	FORGETFULNESS	FEAR OF BEING ALONE
	HEADACHES	
50		LOWER BACK PAIN
	SCIATICA	MULTIPLE ANXIETIES
40	CONFUSION	ASTHMA
	DEFORMED JOINTS	PANIC ATTACKS
30	APATHY - DEPRESSION	
	CONTINUOUS PAIN	UNABLE TO LEAVE HOUSE
20	SUICIDAL THOUGHTS	MUSCLE WEAKNESS
		MULTIPLE SCLEROSIS
10		
0		

the conclusion that these are one and the same disease showing different symptoms. They think each "disease" is a separate process, having its own physiological mechanism, with nothing in common with any other "disease" and therefore they have a different theory for each.

In other words, they think that each "disease" developes in separate and unique ways. The way cancer develops is thought to be entirely different from how diabetes occurs. Multiple sclerosis takes another course altogether. This is like saying that, on a biologic level, an elm tree functions differently than an apple tree. We already know why all our symptoms are related from the examples in previous chapters.

All Nature is based on uniform laws and principles. Conventional medicine is the only area in our world that doesn't subscribe to unifying principles or common natural law that governs all events and processes. It is attempting to understand human health and disease without natural law as its foundation.

Homeopathy has
one theory for all disease and
one mechanism for all symptom development.

There is no fundamental difference between any symptoms, they are all created by the Defense Mechanism. There is no fundamental difference between diseases, they all weaken the Defense Mechanism, necessitating symptoms.

The decline of the Defense Mechanism is not a steady process. You can stay at one level of lowered health for a long time. The symptoms will therefore be constant without progression or remission. Further decline can be caused by a shock, stress or other disease influence. Then, the already compromised Defense Mechanism will be further diminished. Patients, themselves, frequently tell me: "I've never really been well since my father died," "I have never recovered from the birth of my last child" or "This all started after I moved to California." They know very well what it's like to decline a level in health. Very few of us ever have the experience of increasing a level or being restored to a truly healthy state.

What we call the "aging" process is actually
the decline of our Defense Mechanism,
giving us more and more symptoms
as we get older.

Keeping the Defense Mechanism in top running condition is the very best way to stay healthy and "young". We have a good example of this with Hahnemann himself. He had a clear mind and active life for all of his 89 years.

Homeopathy empowers the body to heal itself by improving the functioning of the Defense Mechanism. Before Homeopathic treatment, the Defense Mechanism did not have the power to eliminate the disease. Because the Homeopathic remedy works at the level of the cause, the correct remedy helps the Defense Mechanism become powerful enough to overcome the disease and eliminate it completely. Then and only then, can the Defense Mechanism remove the symptoms it has created.

Disease can be cured only by an improvement in the Defense Mechanism.

Just as disease progression occurs with a reduction in Defense Mechanism activity, the healing process occurs with an increase in its activity. We will show this graphically by a gradual movement up the chart. The Defense Mechanism revisits the same levels of function that it did as it declined in activity.

In our example, we left the patient with a Defense Mechanism activity of 55%. After Homeopathic treatment, the level increases to 65%, a great improvement to start! Remember what the patient's symptoms were at 65% activity. At that level he had a group of symptoms called "pneumonia" which the Defense Mechanism created to restore a balance at that level of disease. Now that he has returned to this level again, he is more susceptible to developing pneumonia than any other symptoms.

The patient is actually in a better state of health than he was before. As bad as pneumonia is, it is much better than the chronic asthma he was experiencing at the level of 55%. The patient continues to improve as the level of the Defense Mechanism improves. As the level increases above 65%, any symptoms from that level also go away.

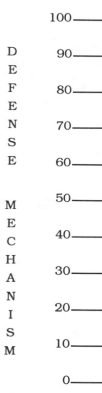

100 — HEALTH

SNEEZING

90 — SORE THROAT, COUGH

80 — BRONCHITIS

70 —

PNEUMONIA

60 —

ASTHMA

50 —

40 —

30 —

20 —

10 —

0 —

DEFENSE MECHANISM

As the level increases to 80%, the bronchitis that occurred earlier at this level could also make an appearance. Conventional medicine always regards bronchitis as "bad" and as an

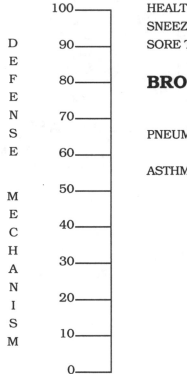

illness requiring treatment. Homeopaths, however, analyze and interpret the bronchitis in terms of what is happening in the whole patient. When the person develops bronchitis, it is not possible to say whether it is a good sign or a bad one unless we know whether the patient had more or less severe symptoms before the bronchitis. If the symptoms were less severe before, then a decline in health is occurring. If the previous symptoms were more severe, then the bronchitis represents an improvement, a movement up the chart. Only after careful evaluation of this entire situation and the patient's whole health history can it be determined if the patient is being restored to health or becoming sicker.

Homeopaths do not just ignore bronchitis or any of the patient's other symptoms. On the contrary, great importance is placed on every symptom and episode. Homeopathy differs from conventional medicine in the analysis and interpretation of what is happening in the entire person, including the Defense Mechanism, the physical body, the mind and the emotions.

Though each of the previous levels will be passed on the way to health, it is not absolutely guaranteed that the symptoms associated with a particular level will come back as that level is revisited. As the patient returns to those specific levels, he is more susceptible to those kinds of symptoms. As he ascends the chart during the healing process, his experience at a specific level is different from when he was getting sicker. The returning symptoms are generally less severe, of shorter duration and better tolerated by the patient as he is getting well.

The Homeopathic remedy is still active in the patient and it continues to improve his Defense Mechanism and his total health. The Defense Mechanism climbs to 90%, 95%, and finally becomes 100% active. Now he is truly cured and totally healthy.

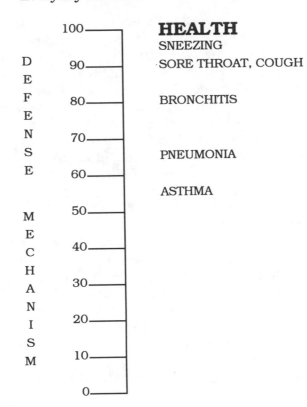

Once the Defense Mechanism has been restored to its full functioning, the patient has then achieved the wonderful level of vitality, freedom and health that is rightfully his as a whole, healthy and joyful human being.

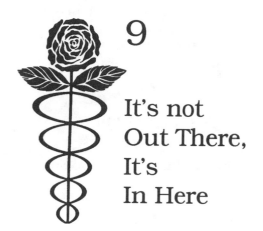

9

It's not
Out There,
It's
In Here

As a general practitioner, I frequently see people with colds, flus and other acute illnesses. These people often think they "caught" their cold from someone at home or at work. Have you ever noticed that in the midst of cold and flu seasons, there are always a few people who don't get sick? It is the strength of their Defense Mechanisms which creates their resistance.

Of course, a person's defense and resistance change as conditions around and in him change. Someone may be well and healthy one day and experience symptoms the next. When this happens his resistance has dropped allowing a disease process to affect him.

Patients often tell me, "This cold has come at the worst possible time! I can't afford to be sick now, I'm too busy." Actually, they have it backward. The cold didn't come at a bad time; it was a bad time, so they got the cold! In almost every case, they were either overworked, not sleeping well or under a tremendous strain of one sort or another all of which lowered their Defense Mechanism's ability to protect them from disease influences.

Remember the times in the past when you developed symptoms. Wasn't it when you were extremely busy, under stress, experiencing strong emotions, overworked, or deprived of enough sleep? A depleted Defense Mechanism allows a disease to be present.

You don't have a disease
because you have symptoms,
you have symptoms
because you have a disease.

Bacteria or other germs are often thought of as the cause of symptoms and disease. We live in a sea of germs, they truly are everywhere! For most of our lives these vast populations of "disease causing agents" don't bother us at all.

When we get "sick", meaning a disease has reduced our Defense Mechanism and its protective boundaries, the germs which are already present, have the opportunity to invade and to participate in the illness. They can't infect unless the Defense Mechanism "invites" them in.

Germs are a secondary result
of a disease process,
not the cause.

In many ways, they are innocent bystanders, waiting for the opportunity to invade. Once they gain a "foot hold", they begin to cause disruptions and additional symptoms. It is our susceptibility or reduced defense that allows them to invade in the first place. A weakened defense always precedes the appearance of the germs and provides them with a favorable environment in which to live. The phrase "catch" a cold is more appropriate than many people realize!

The presence of viruses and bacteria is just one manifestation of an underlying disease process. This is certainly not to say that bacteria, viruses and other microorganisms are all harmless. On the contrary, they can and do disrupt our normal functioning, sometimes in serious and life threatening ways. They rarely can infect a truly healthy person. There must first be a weakness in the Defense Mechanism.

We see this principle often in Nature. In the animal kingdom, it is the animal that is weakened or already ill that is more susceptible to attack, by germs, predators or other animals.

Farley Mohat, a naturalist and biological researcher who spent many years in the wilderness studying wolves, describes this beautifully in his book *Cry Wolf.* Not a particularly popular animal, the wolves' poor reputation was made worse by our general ignorance of their life, habits and ecological niche. They were hated by the people whose livelihood depended on the caribou that the wolves frequently killed for food. Mohat discovered that the only caribou the wolves ever killed were ones that were already diseased. These weakened animals fell easily to an attack while the healthy caribou were simply too fast and strong for the wolves to subdue. Furthermore, he discovered that by killing the afflicted caribou, the wolves actually helped the herd by limiting the spread of disease. Naturally, his research lead to a major change in our opinion and understanding of wolves.

Like the caribou, we must first have a weakened Defense Mechanism before the germs (like the wolves) can overcome us. We can improve our defense, and make our internal environment unfavorable for germs because our body has an innate ability to prevent and cure infections.

Restoring and improving the Defense Mechanism makes it impossible for bacteria and other germs to survive.

Since the discovery of bacteria in the late 1800's, the germ has been thought to be the only factor involved in contagious illness. Whole areas of research, therapeutics and treatment are aimed solely at eliminating the germ, thinking we are thereby eliminating disease. Most of our preventive health measures have been directed at limiting exposure to contagion through hygiene, waste disposal and public sanitation. Whereas these measures have been enormously effective, there has been very little emphasis on decreasing individual susceptibility by improving overall health.

The majority medical opinion is only considering one of the two factors involved in the disease process, the disease strength, ignoring the patient's defense and vulnerability to the infecting agent. To understand where our current ideas came from, let's go back to a time before the invention of microscopes, when bacteria had not yet been discovered.

Naturally, there were theories then too about the cause of disease. Contagion, for example, was thought to be due, in part, to breathing the air in a room where a sick person slept. Divine wrath was also commonly thought to cause disease. There were ideas about the presence of four different "humours" or fluids in the body and disease was thought to result from an imbalance in these fluids. Blood was drained from a patient by cuts or leeches to restore the healthy balance in the four humours. Surgery was virtually unknown, consisting only of amputations or very simple procedures, and then only as a last resort.

It was thought that life could be generated spontaneously from tissue because worms seemed to grow in animal carcasses and in fruit. There were many other ideas, theories and practices that we now, in our self-confident wisdom, look upon with disgust and disdain.

It was against this background that Leewenhowk, a Dutchman who lived between 1632 and 1723, developed and perfected the microscope. This allowed him to discover the world of microorganisms. It was not long before other people began to observe and experiment with the vast array of life forms that had been, until then, hidden from our view and awareness. Over two centuries later, experimental work by Lister, Pasteur and others began to demonstrate the consistent presence of specific micro-organisms in drainage from wounds or in other fluids from the sick.

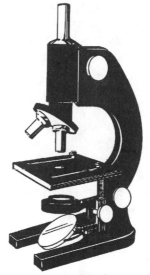

The disease producing effects of microorganisms were further shown by the observation that without a specific germ, expected symptoms did not appear. As surprising as it seems today, the established medical community had enormous resistance to these new ideas about microorganisms and the role they played in disease.

It was the work of a prominent scientist, Robert Koch, that finally succeeded in showing to the scientists' satisfaction that a specific bacteria was actually the cause of a specific disease. In 1876, Koch developed a set of criteria, later known as Koch's postulates, which identify the bacterial "cause of a disease". These criteria are:

1. The bacteria must always be present in the disease.
2. The bacteria can be cultivated outside the infected body.
3. An injection of a pure culture of the bacteria into a healthy animal reproduces the original disease.

Over his lifetime, Koch investigated anthrax, tuberculosis, cholera, malaria and many other diseases. In 1905 he received the Nobel prize in medicine for developing the tuberculin skin test.

The universal adoption of Koch's postulates set the stage for believing that microorganisms alone were responsible for infectious disease. His perspective has been the foundation of our medical system since then. Pasteur, Lister, and others later strengthened this viewpoint. Koch was a brilliant physician and scientist contributing a great deal to medicine. His methods and conclusions, however, left no allowances for individual susceptibility in determining the start of an infectious disease.

Every aspect of mainstream medicine has, as its underlying premise, this idea of a specific biological, mechanical or chemical causative agent which is responsible for a specific "disease". Here I am using the term "disease" as it is generally used in our society; as a name given to a collection of symptoms. Except for a few hereditary diseases, this perspective dominates diagnosis, therapeutics, research and pharmaceuticals.

A good example of this is our current preoccupation with cholesterol levels. Much research has been and continues to be done to learn more about how cholesterol is made and processed in the body. The link between cholesterol and heart disease, arteriosclerosis, vascular disease and other physical problems is being investigated with great fervor. People are now following their cholesterol levels as closely as they follow the stock market, perhaps even more closely.

Many of us have reluctantly changed our dietary habits in the face of the massive evidence published about the influence of diet on cholesterol levels. For some, it seems their bodies do not understand the dangers of an elevated cholesterol level and continue to produce it in what are considered excessive amounts in spite of eliminating cholesterol containing foods from their diet.

Naturally medications, very expensive ones, are now available for those whose cholesterol levels do not meet the new "safe" levels recommended by doctors and scientists. These medications are especially advised for those whose life style or preferences prevent strict adherence to dietary regimes necessary to reduce cholesterol.

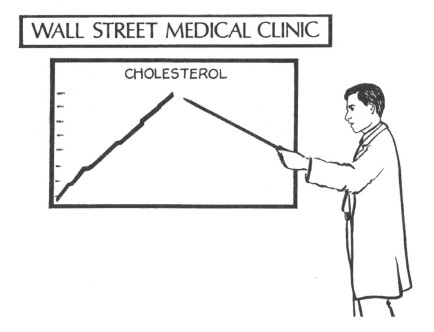

*The forced reduction of cholesterol
by diet or medications
is thought to be of benefit for everyone.*

The majority of the evidence condemning cholesterol comes from a very narrow perspective on the issue. Most research studies don't consider other aspects of a persons' life, health and temperament when evaluating the role of cholesterol in the formation of arteriosclerosis. In fact, they purposely eliminate all other factors except the cholesterol level itself! How can the researchers be sure that these other factors are unimportant? Is it possible that ignoring these factors is also limiting the possibilities for a valuable discovery?

There are still many unanswered questions. For example, why do some people tolerate high cholesterol levels while others do not? Why do dietary restrictions of cholesterol work to lower the blood levels in some people and not in others? To fully understand the impact of cholesterol, diet and disease we must incorporate internal factors and individual differences in our research.

One particularly interesting study, published in the prestigious magazine, Science, in June 1980, proves this point. This study describes the development of arteriosclerosis in rabbits fed a high cholesterol diet. No surprise here.

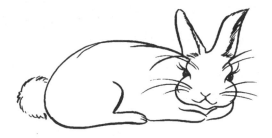

What is a surprise is that one group of rabbits showed a 60% decrease in severity and occurrence of arteriosclerosis as compared to the other rabbits. This special group was petted, played with and cuddled as part of their daily routine. The other rabbits did not receive this extra care and attention.

There was no significant difference in the cholesterol levels of the two groups yet the special group formed significantly less arteriosclerosis. This example shows arteriosclerosis to be independent of the amount of cholesterol eaten or the level of cholesterol in the blood. This is a revolutionary idea and contrary to conventional medical thought.

This study points to the major role that non-dietary, social, emotional and other factors could have in our overall health. These findings have great significance for those of us who are interested in our cholesterol level and its true role in disease. Despite the relevance of these factors, few of the major clinical studies of the past or those currently underway consider our emotions, character, job satisfaction, or the nature of our personal relationships and the impact these factors have on vascular disease formation.

Certainly more research needs to be done. If life style, temperament, emotions and other difficult to quantify elements do have a profound effect on the development of arteriosclerosis, then these elements should be considered and included in the design of current cholesterol research and interpretation of results.

There is another great problem with retaining the conventional, exclusively physical, mechanistic view of the human being. This approach to diagnosis and treatment distracts us from looking in the right places for the true cure of disease.

We are still looking "OUT THERE"
in the environment
for the reasons we have symptoms,
rather than "IN HERE",
our overall health and defense against disease.

If we are convinced that cholesterol is the cause of arteriosclerosis, then reducing serum cholesterol by diet or medication seems the best way to prevent that problem. We are also not likely to look beyond that point to the other factors that also may prevent arteriosclerosis.

Let's look at the issue of cholesterol and arteriosclerosis from the perspective of Homeopathy. In chapter three, we talked about the causative pathways leading to arthritis and hypertension. Remember that both elevated cholesterol and arteriosclerosis are symptoms and are therefore developed, as are all symptoms, by the Defense Mechanism in an effort to counteract an inner disease process. If we treat only the symptoms of cholesterol level or arteriosclerosis and not the true underlying cause, the disease process will remain active.

Simply lowering our cholesterol will not cure us.

Fortunately, we have Homeopathy which not only looks at cholesterol, and arteriosclerosis but also considers emotions, life-style, temperament, job satisfaction and most importantly, individual susceptibility to disease. It should not surprise you that when these aspects are included in patient evaluation and treatment, the patient's health improves dramatically .

We have found that illness is not so much a result of what is "out there" as it is a result of what is "in here". Both factors, the strength of the disease influence (outside) and the strength of the Defense Mechanism (inside) determine if we get sick. Any medical system that is truly going to improve our lives and cure our diseases must look inside us as well as outside.

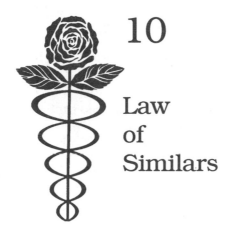

10

Law
of
Similars

As a scientific system of medicine, Homeopathy is governed by the same physical laws and biologic principles that govern all other aspects of nature and the world around us. Some of the biologic principles involved in Homeopathy may not be familiar to you.

The fundamental principle on which Homeopathy is based is called the Law of Similars, which comes from the Latin *Similia Similibus Curentur*, meaning "Like cures Like". The term "Homeopathy", literally translated from the Greek, means "same sickness", which also refers to the Law of Similars.

The Law of Similars states that when a healthy person ingests a substance, a plant or mineral perhaps, certain distinct symptoms appear. Whenever a sick person has those same symptoms, he will be cured by taking that substance in Homeopathic form.

The Law of Similars is
the great secret of true healing.

This amazing concept is made even more remarkable by its divergence from standard medical thought. It is, none the less, a biologic fact and has been demonstrated and used in healing for centuries.

Hippocrates (460 - 370 B.C.), known as the father of medicine, was possibly the first to record this concept of healing. A prolific writer about a variety of aspects in medicine, he recorded many cases in which he observed that the medicine known to cause a problem, could also cure that same problem. Galen (200 - 130 B.C.), whose teachings dominated medical thought for over 1600 years, also observed instances which verified the Law of Similars.   Paracelsus (1493-1541), the controversial medical genius of the middle ages, knew of and used this principle. The Arabs in southern Spain also may have had knowledge of this principle and used it in their extensive medical system when Europe was still in the Dark Ages.

Although the Law of Similars was known all this time, it wasn't put to practical use in a medical system of therapeutics until the late 1700's when Samuel Hahnemann, MD developed Homeopathy.

Dr. Hahnemann's journey toward the discovery of Homeopathy began with his extensive knowledge of the medicinal properties of plants and other natural substances.   As a physician he had first hand knowledge of the effects of these botanical medicines.   He also spent many years translating classic texts on chemistry, biology, physics, medicine and other scientific subjects. This introduced him to a variety of aspects of disease processes as described by other physicians, both ancient and contemporary to him. All this lead him to perceive and apply the workings of the Law of Similars.

The study of malaria began the use of the Law of Similars in a medical system. In Hahnemann's time, malaria was a very common and devastating disease.   It was treated by the administration of cinchona bark which contains the active ingredient quinine. Our treatment today, to a large extent, still involves quinine.   It was Hahnemann's brilliant observation that the symptoms of malaria and the symptoms of quinine poisoning are the same. This was Hahnemann's first experience that symptoms of a disease are cured by ingesting the same medicine that produces those symptoms in a healthy person.

Not content with the observations of others, Hahnemann took quinine himself to see what symptoms would develop; they were identical to malaria. Soon the symptoms subsided and he was well again. This experience gave him a profound insight into the nature of disease process and therapeutics. Thanks to Hahnemann's inquiring, observing nature and his dedication to truth, he did not just leave this observation to be buried by the prominent medical philosophy of his day.

Hahnemann began his life's work, the development of Homeopathy.

There was a large amount of recorded knowledge about the effects of many substances on the human body. Hahnemann already knew distinct sets of symptoms produced by many substances which could theoretically cure illness. He continued his observations to see if these substances would cure the symptoms they produced in a healthy person just as quinine had. His experiments showed that these other substances did indeed cure as predicted by the Law of Similars.

Many substances that were needed therapeutically were, themselves, very poisonous. Since no other substances could be found that produced those specific symptoms, Hahnemann had to find a way to make them safe for use in treatment. He reduced the dose of the medicine to extremely small, dilute quantities. By doing this, Hahnemann found that the toxic effects of the medicine were eliminated while its curative action remained.

With the removal of toxic and dangerous properties of substances through dilution, the number of natural products that could be used medicinally expanded enormously. In fact, substances that are the most poisonous in their natural state often become the most useful Homeopathic medicines.

Most of us have experienced the Law of Similars in action. At sometime or another, we all have chopped an onion or at least we have been close enough to this process to experience the unpleasant sensations of burning, stinging eyes with lots of tearing. According to the Law of Similars, someone having those symptoms without being exposed to an onion should be cured by an onion. This is exactly what happens in practice.

Hayfever sufferers will recognize these symptoms immediately! Indeed, onion is one of the best remedies for the relief of hayfever. I'm not suggesting that you go to your local market and get an onion to alleviate your hayfever. That would certainly make you worse! Only the Homeopathic preparation of onion will cure you. Though this example is an external exposure to the onion instead of ingestion, the Law of Similars still applies.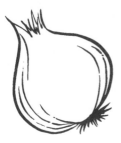

An example from the conventional medical world shows that the Law of Similars works even when it isn't recognized. Conventional medicine uses a drug called digoxin (Lanoxin) for treatment of a variety of heart problems. This wonderfully effective medication comes from the foxglove plant and has been used for centuries as a heart tonic. It is so effective in the treatment of certain types of irregular heart beat and atrial fibrillation, that it is still used today as a preferred treatment for those conditions. Due to its toxicity, caution is needed when administering digoxin because of its potential for causing serious problems.

One of the conditions successfully treated by digoxin is atrial fibrillation. When a patient suffers from this condition, the top portion of the heart, the atria, trembles instead of beating regularly. The blood is not forced naturally into the lower part of the heart, the ventricles. The heart then can't effectively pump the blood from the ventricles into the body. Both the slow discharge of blood from the atria and the irregular and inefficient beating of the ventricles cause many problems in all areas of the body.

After the patient takes digoxin, the atria beat normally and the ventricles, which now have blood delivered in the usual way, also function normally. So far this sounds like standard conventional treatment. Where does Homeopathy and the Law of Similars come in?

According to the Law of Similars, when a healthy person takes a substance it will produce the same symptoms that the substance can cure in a sick person. What symptoms would you expect when a healthy person takes digoxin? Exactly! The person develops atrial fibrillation and irregular heart beats appear.

In fact, the symptoms of overdose with digoxin or foxglove are so similar to the symptoms it treats that many intentional and undetected poisonings have been committed with this drug. The unfortunate victims were mistakenly thought to have died of the natural consequences of their heart problems. In mystery stories, many tiresome spouses have died of "accidental" overdoses of their required foxglove administered by their "loving" partners!

Once a patient has had his normal heart rhythm restored by digoxin, taking more of the drug again produces atrial fibrillation, just as it would if a healthy person took it. This observation was made years ago by the conventional medical community and is the basis for the extreme caution exercised by all doctors when administering digoxin. Conventional medical doctors say that digoxin will "cause the same disease that it can cure." That sure sounds like the Law of Similars to me.

Homeopaths know that there are other times, besides atrial fibrillation, when a patient needs digoxin. For example, this Homeopathic remedy can be used for an enlargement of the liver due to heart problems, for a weakness in the stomach with tenderness, or for certain urinary and prostate problems. How did we learn all this about digoxin?

Hahnemann learned much about the usual medical indications for digoxin and other plants, minerals and natural substances from the observations and experience of physicians who were knowledgeable about their use. Other useful information came from records of accidental poisonings. All this information was compiled in books called Herbals which were among the resources for physicians of that time. Previous generations relied exclusively on botanical and other natural sources for their medicines. Only recently has the pharmaceutical industry provided medicines that were newly created or purified in the laboratory instead of coming directly from nature.

Most of what we know about the medicinal actions of Homeopathic substances was discovered by Hahnemann himself and later by his followers. According to the Law of Similars, Hahnemann knew that giving a substance to a healthy person would produce the same set of symptoms that it could cure. So this is exactly what he did. In a process called "proving", Hahnemann and later his students, followers and others ingested small amounts of single substances. They kept extremely detailed and accurate notes of their experiences, physical symptoms, thoughts, reactions and sensations. The symptoms the substance produced would be the ones that it could cure as a Homeopathic remedy. It is this first hand experience, how an individual remedy actually works in the human being, which makes Homeopathy an extremely precise and accurate medical system.

Hahnemann, himself, proved almost 100 substances. Others would later add to that number so that today there are about 2000 tested substances used as Homeopathic remedies.

All the information collected from the provings has been complied into books called Materia Medicas. These books often include clinical experience about the patient's symptoms that consistently went away after using a specific Homeopathic remedy. Provings followed by clinical experience has been the mainstay of Homeopathic knowledge, providing the firm foundation on which Homeopaths worldwide have relied for two centuries.

Each Homeopath must learn and understand all the ways each remedy affects the human being. Not only do these remedies produce physical symptoms but also emotional and mental ones. All those effects make up the entire set of symptoms known for that remedy and indicate the illnesses and symptoms it will relieve.

The mental and emotional symptoms associated with the individual remedies are particularly interesting. We often believe that thoughts and personality characteristics are ours alone and that we have ultimate control over them. These characteristics and thoughts are as much a part of our overall state of health and disease as any other symptom. Anger, jealousy, irritability, punctuality, excitement, ambition, laziness, honesty, cruelty, combativeness, introversion, timidity, flamboyance, sensuality, depression, industriousness and thousands of other attributes can and will change for the better after Homeopathic treatment.

Through decades of careful and accurate observation by Homeopaths, we now know that every patient's symptoms fall into very predictable and precise sets or constellations that exactly match the symptom sets produced by the individual Homeopathic remedies. As the Defense Mechanism declines in strength, the symptoms it creates will match those of a single remedy which has demonstrated the ability to cure that particular set of symptoms.

Symptoms always occur in constellations that are represented by a specific Homeopathic remedy.

The information about many individual remedies is very complete and includes descriptions of the emotions, character and personality. This enables a Homeopath to understand a great deal about the patient. For example, when a patient's physical complaint is cured by a certain remedy, it is possible to know something about his character. Conversely, knowing the character, I will know the physical symptoms for which he is at risk. Specific personality characteristics are associated with distinct physical problems as predicted by the remedy and its complete constellation of symptoms.

In recent years, conventional medical doctors have become aware of the connection between certain personality types and specific medical problems. The hard-driving, ambitious work-a-holic or so-called "Type A" personality is known to be at great risk for ulcers, hypertension and indigestion. Homeopaths have understood this and many other personality-physical symptom connections for nearly 200 years!

Each remedy has unique characteristics which lead a Homeopath to the correct remedy even when he doesn't know all the patient's symptoms. Once the appropriate Homeopathic remedy is given, all the symptoms go away even if they were not originally discussed with the Homeopath. Often a patient will return to my office, enthusiastically reporting the improvement of a particularly annoying symptom, only to discover he had neglected to even mention it in the first interview! It is the Homeopath's job is find the correct remedy for the patient. The remedy will do the rest.

As an example, suppose it is your job to identify a certain painting. You are allowed only one guess and your payment depends on how quickly and accurately you can do the job. When you first see the painting, it is covered by a cloth that hides it from view.

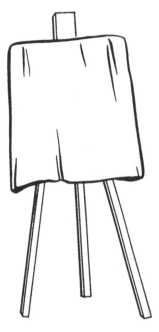

At selected time intervals the cloth moves, revealing an additional small portion of the painting. You want to make your guess as quickly as possible to get the highest payment, but you also must wait until you can see enough of the painting to ensure your accuracy.

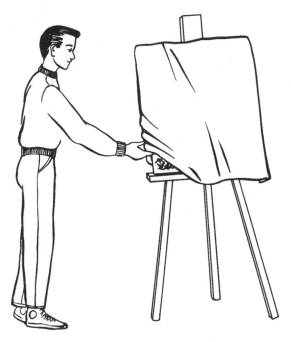

Once the revealed area of the painting has provided just enough information to identify it accurately, you will be absolutely sure what the rest of the painting looks like.

What matters most, is the identification, not how much information you collect to accomplish it.

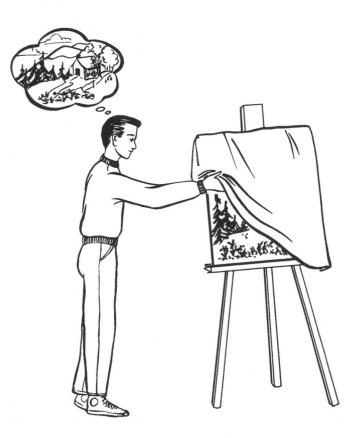

This is very much like the Homeopath's job of identifying the one appropriate remedy for a patient. The Homeopath must collect just enough information to prescribe the correct remedy. Once that remedy has been identified, no further information is needed. This sometimes leaves patients with the impression that they have not said enough about their symptoms. The goal is to choose the right remedy and all questioning is aimed solely at that purpose.

When a patient complains, "I have a headache" they are giving very little information. Any one of several hundred different Homeopathic remedies could be the right one. After careful questioning and observation to discover additional details of the symptoms and clues to the patient's overall condition, a very clear, three dimensional picture or image of the patient in his current state becomes evident. This constellation of symptoms matches those of a specific remedy, for example, Natrum muriaticum. When the patient takes this remedy, the headaches and any other symptoms, will go away.

To tell a Homeopath that the patient has a diagnosis of "headache" also conveys very little useful information. To say, however, that the patient is in a disease state requiring a specific remedy, Natrum muriaticum in this case, gives the Homeopath an enormous amount of detail about the condition of the whole person. Having Materia Medicas as reference books with such unique and detailed information about individual remedies, makes this system of disease and symptom identification much more accurate.

Homeopaths describe illness and make diagnoses in terms of remedy names. I refer to the disease state of the patient by the name of the particular remedy that will eliminate that state and restore the patient to health. Using the same name for both the disease and remedy that cures it can be confusing. For example, a person needing Pulsatilla to cure them would be in a Pulsatilla state. The disease is named Pulsatilla and so is the remedy they need.

There are over 2000 different Homeopathic remedies. Is it possible that all illnesses and varieties of human beings fall into only 2000 categories? Can Homeopathic treatment be so individualized if there is only a limited number of remedies? Yes it can! The therapeutic range of the Homeopathic remedies is tremendous.

Not every symptom a remedy is capable of producing (and curing) will be present in a patient needing that remedy for treatment. A patient will rarely, if ever, have all those symptoms. Only a small number of the total possible symptoms are usually evident. These are enough, however, to identify the correct remedy. Each remedy (disease state) can present itself through combinations of its symptoms in a limitless number of ways. This accounts for the enormous variety of human conditions that can be treated with a limited number of Homeopathic remedies.

The patient does not need to have all the symptoms of the remedy, however, the remedy must have all the symptoms of the patient.

In the example of the onion, the hayfever patient only had symptoms in the eyes. From the Materia Medica we know that onion (Allium cepa) also effects other areas including the stomach, intestines and respiratory system. None of these other symptoms were present and were not needed to prescribe Allium cepa. When it is the appropriate remedy, Allium cepa will work even if only one or any combination of its specific characteristics are present. The patient was in an "Allium cepa" state and therefore, Allium cepa cured the whole patient.

A remedy, such as Calcarea carbonica, can produce its characteristic symptoms in every area of the body, mind and emotions. Here the circle represents *all* the symptoms that Calcarea carbonica can produce and, therefore, cure.

One patient requiring Calcarea carbonica may only show a problem in the lungs with shortness of breath. Another patient may have eczema and sleeplessness while another may have panic attacks and a stomach disorder. They all, however, have some symptoms and characteristics in common; chilly temperature and sugar cravings. These divergent manifestations are all possible in the Calcarea carbonica state and will be treated successfully with that remedy and no other. By evaluating each of these patients and collecting a thorough list of all their symptoms and characteristics, the Homeopath will see that Calcarea carbonica is the correct remedy, despite the differences in their presenting complaints.

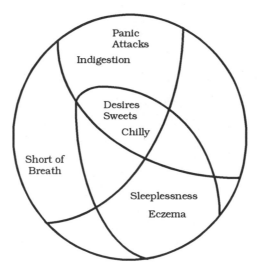

CALCAREA CARBONICA

Each person's Defense Mechanism, their hierarchy of symptoms, their constitutional characteristics and the extent of their disease process all play a role in how and where symptoms will first appear and which symptoms out of the total possible for that remedy will be developed at any given time.

In chapter eight, we used graphs to show susceptibility and states of health. The interaction of the Defense Mechanism and the disease determines the level of health. The hierarchy of symptoms combined with the specific characteristics of a particular remedy determine exactly what symptoms are present at any level. We can redraw the graph to show that the decline in health and resulting symptoms follows the symptom patterns of an individual remedy.

```
              100 ─────┐       HEALTH

   D           90 ─────┤       ECZEMA
   E
   F           80 ─────┤       INDIGESTION
   E                           HEARTBURN
   N           70 ─────┤       BLOATING
   S                           IRRITABLE
   E           60 ─────┤
                               GALLSTONES
                50 ─────┤       EXTENSIVE ECZEMA
   M                           ANXIETIES
   E           40 ─────┤
   C
   H           30 ─────┤       ARTHRITIS
   A                           ALCOHOLISM
   N
   I           20 ─────┤
   S
   M           10 ─────┤

                0 ─────┘
```

Symptoms of one remedy changing as a disease progresses is called remedy "stages". During the initial disease process, only a few minor symptoms are needed. Later, as the disease advances, these early symptoms go away and are replaced by others of a more significant nature. All the symptoms, however, are from the same remedy. The same remedy also will produce different sets of symptoms in children, adolescents, adults and the elderly.

How does the correct remedy actually work to cure a person? There are several things we already know. When a person is ill, he will exhibit a set of symptoms. The symptoms are specifically picked by the Defense Mechanism to restore balance. The Defense Mechanism and the disease influence are fairly evenly matched. If the defense was stronger than the disease influence, no symptoms would have appeared and if the disease had been very much stronger than the Defense Mechanism, then death would have resulted.

*Symptoms indicate that
the Defense Mechanism is trying,
but is not quite able,
to overcome the disease force and eliminate it.*

The symptoms are the Defense Mechanism's best effort to combat and compensate for the disease force. The precision with which the Defense Mechanism creates the symptoms is a sign of its wisdom in knowing exactly what is needed to counteract the disease.

In the following diagram, the arrow on the right signifies the disease with its specific "shape" and strength. The Defense Mechanism will exactly counteract this disease force with it's arrow, which is on the left. It's shape represents the different symptoms that the Defense Mechanism produces to counteract the disease influence precisely.

Both arrows are of equal strength, thereby preventing either the disease or the defense from completely overpowering the other.

The Defense Mechanism has already determined the kind of symptoms needed to fight the disease; there is no need for additional symptoms. It just doesn't have the strength to produce them with enough power. It needs greater strength of the symptoms that are already present to overcome the disease

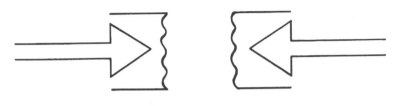

DEFENSE MECHANISM   DISEASE

influence and end the need for those symptoms. If only the Defense Mechanism had just a little more power!

By taking a Homeopathic remedy that has proven it can produce those exact symptoms, the Defense Mechanism is given that extra power. From the remedy it gets a little bit more of what it has already shown it needs to fight the disease and overpower it. Graphically, the arrow shaft has grown wider.

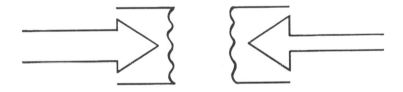

Now that the disease is eliminated, the symptoms are no longer needed and they disappear. You can see in the illustration that the arrow is now uncovered.

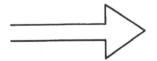

Homeopathic treatment involves discovering which symptoms the patient's Defense Mechanism has already produced and then giving the specific remedy that is known to create those same symptoms. It can be as straight forward as matching the symptoms cured by the remedy to the symptoms in the patient, using the Law of Similars. While this may seem simple, any Homeopath will tell you that it is far from easy. Now you can understand why good Homeopathic prescribing is difficult and quite complex despite being based on the simple principle expressed in the Law of Similars.

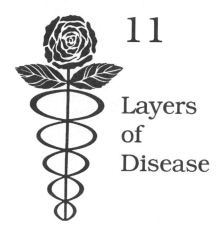

11

Layers of Disease

Symptoms come and go, problems change from one area to another, disease advances and defense retreats, defense improves and disease recoils. There's a lot of commotion going on in us and amidst all this flurry of activity, symptoms are always being created to maintain and restore the needed balance.

The natural progression of a disease and deterioration of the Defense Mechanism are not the only reasons why additional symptoms appear. New disease influences, conventional medical treatment or suppression of symptoms all result in a greater intensity of existing symptoms and the creation of new ones.

A series of symptoms change from one to another. If the path they take is distinctly characteristic for a single specific remedy, then only that remedy will be needed to help the patient. Often another disease influence comes in and upsets the balance again, which necessitates the creation of even more symptoms. These new symptoms may indicate that a different remedy is needed. The path has changed directions due to a layering of disease.

To illustrate this idea of the layers of disease let's use a table with three table cloths on it. The first cloth on the table is embroidered with lace on the edges.   This represents the healthy state. As you can see, two more tablecloths are placed on top.

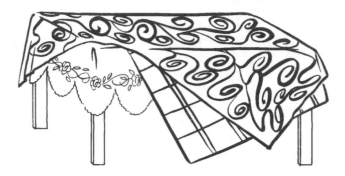

Our patient, the table, seeks Homeopathic treatment saying "You know, doctor, I just don't feel well, something isn't right. I used to do so much and now I'm always tired. I can hardly get to work anymore and I don't seem to care about anything except sitting around.   I just don't know what it is."

The symptoms a patient expresses are needed to guide the Homeopath to the correct remedy. Unfortunately, the symptoms so far are rather nonspecific and vague.   It is up to the Homeopath to question the patient, observe him and gather as much information as possible.

The whole person always gives
enough information
to the Homeopath to prescribe correctly.
He must have
the perception and wisdom to see it.

In a Homeopathic interview, we investigate the exact details of all the symptoms. Typically, this starts with the main complaint. The Homeopath also notes the emotional state, food preferences, sleep patterns, family, social and work situations and experiences, certain aspects of the patient's character and how he reacts to specific kinds of stresses and many other kinds of information. The Homeopath observes the patient's appearance, tone of voice, style of dress, manner of answering questions and other non-verbal clues. It can sometimes take two hours to gather enough information from these areas before the correct remedy can be prescribed.

Let's play Homeopathic sleuth and see what other information we can gather by observing and describing our "patient". He has a flat top, with black swirls which are somewhat wrinkled. Have you ever had that wrinkled feeling? I know I have! On the side there is a triangular area of black and white checks. The patient has four legs, is cool to the touch and is a bit wobbly. We can see a little bit of lace and embroidery showing. This is quite a list of symptoms in addition to those directly expressed by the patient.

All of these symptoms tell us that our patient is not in a very healthy state! With the list of symptoms completed, our next step is to use it to choose a remedy based on the Law of Similars. We will read through the Materia Medica looking for the remedy that most closely represents the whole constellation of symptoms presented.

In referring to the Materia Medica, we have discovered a remedy that can cure black swirls, can stop that wrinkled feeling, can improve temperature and is also well known for its helpful effect on wobbliness. This addresses quite a few of the patient's main symptoms. Before prescribing this remedy we will thoroughly check the Materia Medica to be sure that there isn't another remedy that has an even closer match to the whole set of symptoms. When we are certain that the most accurate remedy has been located, we will prescribe it for the patient.

What happens next? The symptoms treated by this remedy disappear. The top table cloth has now been removed.

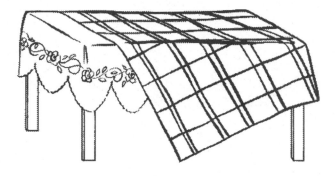

In many cases, one remedy, carefully prescribed, will bring a patient back to his healthy, balanced state of joyful, vital health. This indicates that all the symptoms, past and present, are related to that single remedy.

Our patient, however, isn't well yet. He returns to us in about six months and reports "I feel so much better! In fact, I feel great. I don't have that wrinkled feeling and I'm not so cool any more. Overall I am greatly improved. There is one problem, though. Do you remember that little bit of black and white check that I had? After taking the remedy, it got much bigger and it is really starting to bother me alot. The funny thing about it is that I used to have this same thing a long time ago but it went away just about the time I got the swirls. Now it's back again. Can you do anything about it?"

As Homeopaths, we know that the return of old symptoms can be a very good sign for two reasons. First, it shows that the remedy is acting to increase the strength of the Defense Mechanism and is moving the patient to a healthier state, "up the graph" of health discussed in chapter eight. Secondly, this can signify that a layer of illness has been removed. Here, the initial remedy has eliminated the effects of the most recent disease influence, the black swirls. Instead of being totally cured, another previous disease state, which caused the black and white checks, can now express itself.

When a disease affects a person, a set of symptoms developes. Later, if another disease influence affects them, a new and different set of symptoms may be required. Only the symptoms from the most recent disease state can be present and all symptoms are related to that disease.

We can have only ONE disease at a time.

Symptoms from a previous disease state will be "covered up" by the existence of the new disease and its symptoms.

Accumulated disease states are similar to a stack of trays in a cafeteria. Only one tray is visible at a time. Put a tray on the stack, and it pushes down the previous tray. The process of healing these different disease states is like pulling the top tray off. The tray underneath immediately pops up and is ready to be pulled off. This process continues until all the trays have been removed. When the correct Homeopathic remedy is given and the top disease layer is removed, then and only then, can the next layer with its distinct symptoms appear and respond to treatment.

The symptom of black and white checks appeared as the swirls went away. In a sense, this symptom was literally covered over by the newer symptom, the swirls. As the healing progresses, the most recent symptoms will be cured first, allowing for the reappearance of a previous state and its symptoms.

As a disease advances, symptoms progress from the least troublesome to more serious. Therefore, when a patient is being cured and goes back through these states in reverse order, the returning symptoms are usually less serious.

Though there may be a return of a previous state, that does

not mean that the patient must suffer with those symptoms. The Homeopath approaches this situation in a way that is similar to the first patient visit. He again questions, observes and lists the patient's symptoms and then refers to the original list of symptoms to note the changes that have occurred since the first treatment.

For our "patient" there have been several changes. The swirls, wobbliness, coldness and wrinkled feelings have now been eliminated. There are also symptoms which are unchanged: the four legs, flat top, lace and embroidered edge. We also must look for the return of old symptoms, new symptoms or increased intensity of current symptoms. Instead of a small triangle of black and white checks, a large area has now appeared. This shows that an old symptom has returned.

After revising the list of symptoms, the Homeopath analyzes the new situation. If the symptom constellation still matches the remedy previously given, then the patient already has the correct remedy he needs to get well. Sometimes just an additional dose of this same remedy is needed. If, however, this set of symptoms doesn't match the previous remedy, then a new prescription is needed. If that is the case, the Homeopath again searches the Materia Medica for a remedy that will cure these symptoms. The decision about what to prescribe and when can only be made after a thorough evaluation of the patient and his current symptoms.

In this case, the "patient's" symptoms do not match the description given in the Materia Medica for the first remedy. They do match another remedy, so that one is now prescribed.

The "patient" experiences a dramatic change after taking the new remedy. The black and white checks disappear.

Now what is left? The formerly small area of cloth with lace and embroidery now covers the whole table top. This is the true state of health for the table and the way it was before any disease layers began. There are still four legs and a flat top. Those things are just an inherent part of being a table. Homeopathy isn't ever going to change that.

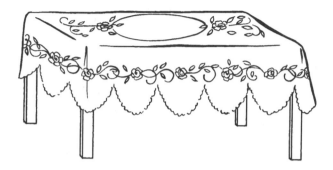

Homeopathy doesn't make us all the same.
It helps you be a better "you"!

This kind of thorough cure is available to you now. It isn't necessary to accept anything less.

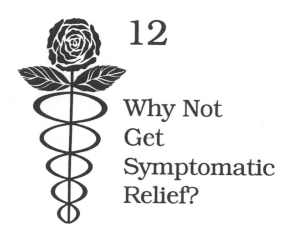

12

Why Not
Get
Symptomatic
Relief?

I'm sure you would like to remain as healthy as possible and would do anything necessary to help maintain a vital, healthy, optimally functioning Defense Mechanism.

Most of us, however, are continually doing things that disrupt, disturb, hinder and compromise the actions of our Defense Mechanism. How is it that our desire to assist our own health actually speeds up the deterioration of the very part of us that protects us from disease?

There is widespread lack of genuine understanding of just how the Defense Mechanism works and the vital role that symptoms play in the preservation of balance within us. Symptoms are typically considered the "enemy" which needs to be conquered. Every attempt is made to eliminate them as quickly as possible through medications, surgery or other therapies.

Rarely do we realize that symptoms are created by the Defense Mechanism in a very precise way to compensate for an internal disease process. They are seldom, if ever, regarded as important signals and guides for the identification of the disease and therefore instrumental in finding the appropriate cure.

As we have seen, conventional medicine regards symptoms as the disease itself, rather than the effects of the disease. From this perspective, the elimination or disappearance of selected symptoms would represent a cure. This symptom oriented approach to medical treatment has created several problems, including leaving the cause of the symptoms untreated. Let's use the following scenario as an illustration.

Suppose that you found a small spot of mildew in the center of your living room wall.

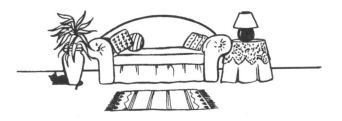

What would you do? Would you tear down the wall to find the source of the mildew, the dampness itself? Not likely! If you took that step, it would require putting up a new wall, painting the entire room and then applying new wallpaper. Like most of us, you would probably just put a picture over the mildew. After all, it's just a little spot.

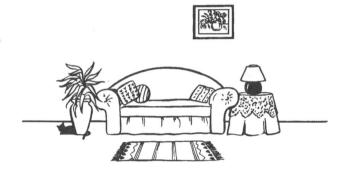

The mildew continues to grow. Eventually, it outgrows the picture you used to hide it.

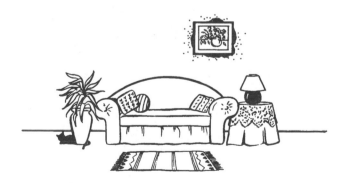

Now, you need a larger picture.

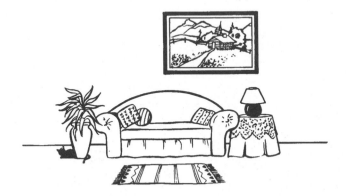

This hides the spot for a while longer.   Finally, the spot grows so large, you can't put a picture over it.

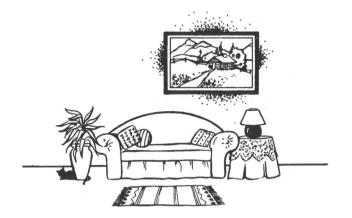

At that point, you must wallpaper the entire area to cover it up.

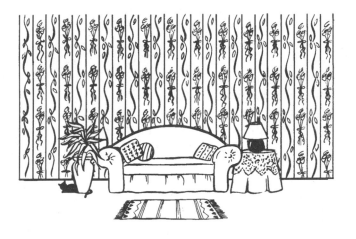

Though you have been successful at hiding the visible mildew, the destruction inside the wall continues. Imagine your surprise when the wall eventually falls down!

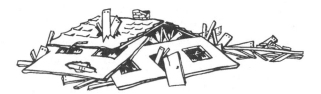

The cause of the mildew was not eliminated, the mildew was only covered up. The symptom was hidden, yet the problem continued. The effect was changed or disguised but the cause remained. Maybe you weren't always aware of it, but it was still there. Obviously, if you had fixed the wall by eliminating the dampness in the very beginning, instead of merely covering up the problem, the inevitable extensive destruction would have been completely avoided. Initially, it seems like a lot to replace part of the wall when only a small spot of mildew is present, however, we can see that ignoring the problem is much more destructive and costly.

Illness works in the same way. When an illness starts, typically only minor symptoms are produced. Generally we either ignore them or simply take mild, non-prescription medication. For example, if you have a runny nose and are sneezing, you might take an antihistamine. This is just the same as putting the picture over the spot on the wall. The real cause is ignored or disguised but it is still very active and will continue to produce more serious symptoms later.

The real solution to the problem of the mildew on the wall is to get rid of the cause by removing all the dampness. Homeopathy is also a real solution because it rids the body of the disease, which is causing the symptoms.

Those small, seemingly "meaningless" symptoms are the signals from the Defense Mechanism that a disease is present and needs to be cured just as the spot of mildew alerted you to an underlying problem in the wall.   While conventional medications generally do give immediate symptomatic relief they also ensure the production of more dangerous and debilitating problems from an untreated, growing disease.

This is another major difference between conventional medicine and Homeopathic medicine. Conventional treatment with its emphasis on individual symptoms, only treats the effects of the disease.   On the other hand, Homeopathic treatment cures because it treats and eliminates the disease itself.

As an example of how our Defense Mechanism works, we used a climate controlled high-rise office building and its central processing station which works to maintain the "healthy state" of the building. Carrying this example further, we can gain even more understanding of the difference between the symptom-oriented and the cause-oriented approach to treating disease.

As you recall, the climate controlled building with its central processing station maintains many parameters in a constant range for the comfort of the inhabitants and for the

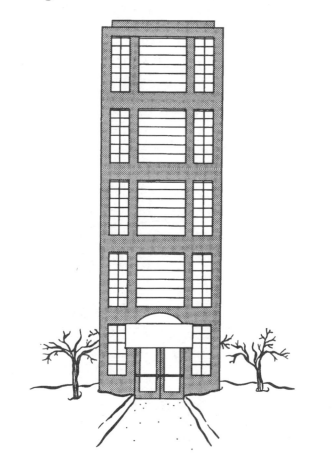

efficient and smooth operation of the building. The central station, like the Defense Mechanism, senses, adjusts, compensates and controls these important parameters. Any alteration in the environment results in the appropriate adjustment. As long as the adjustment required is within the capabilities of the central processing station, everything runs very smoothly.

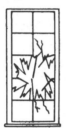

Sometimes things happen that are beyond the central processing station's ability to maintain equilibrium. For example, a window in the front entry gets broken. During winter, the temperature in this area drops quickly.

Even without detecting the cause, the central station detects the drop in temperature and makes the usual adjustments. The furnace tries to reheat the building. This is not possible as long as the window is broken, so the temperature remains low.

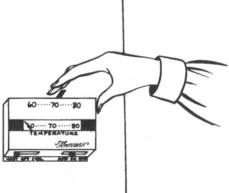

The people, now uncomfortable with the persistent lower temperature, assume that something is wrong with the thermostat and turn it up. They don't realize that the thermostat is working correctly and that the real problem is the broken window. The "symptom" is the drop in temperature, the "disease" is the broken window.

Reheating the building isn't a very efficient way to handle the situation. It makes more sense to "cure" the cause by replacing the window. For now the heat has been turned up in an effort to maintain a comfortable temperature. By trying to handle the problem in this way, other "symptoms" are likely to occur.

For example, the utility bills will increase dramatically. When the manager gets the bill, he immediately becomes aware that there must be something very wrong within the building.

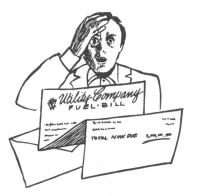

A few phone calls, or a visit to the building reveals the problem. Now the curative approach is taken and the broken window is replaced. The central processing station will detect that the temperature is now within the acceptable range and no extra heat is needed.

We can see the difference between treating the cause and treating the effect. The central processing station, like our Defense Mechanism, did what it was designed to do; it detected a change, the drop in temperature, and then made every attempt within its capabilities to correct the situation. It cannot correct the "cause" by replacing the window; that required help from an outside service. The symptom of an enormous fuel bill, created by the efforts of the central processing station to do its job, was the signal that alerted the manager that there was a "disease" situation that had overpowered the central station's abilities. The central station could not correct the cause of the problem itself but it did create enough "symptoms" to draw attention to the cause and get it fixed.

Let's look at a different scenario, one which relates to the times when we ignore symptoms. For some reason, the manager never sees the heating bill or ignores it. Using some imagination, we can predict what might happen. The furnace, not designed to heat a lobby with a large broken window during winter, will eventually malfunction. The staff in the reception area begins to get sick. They develop colds, bronchitis or even pneumonia.

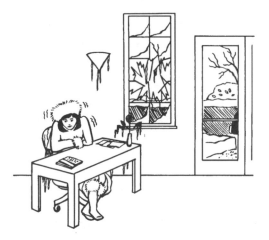

The enormous cost of the fuel deprives other areas in the building of operating funds. The security guards won't be paid and they will quit. There won't be enough money for electricity. These and other problems would affect every aspect of the entire building. Eventually the initial cause, the broken window, will result in such deterioration that it could cause closure of the building or bankruptcy of the owners. This may seem extreme and very unlikely but drawing out the example to this conclusion shows how severe and complicated problems can become from one initial cause.

Of course, all this directly applies to how we function as human beings. When an influence from the environment is too great for our Defense Mechanism to withstand, a disease process starts. Our Defense Mechanism will try to restore balance by compensating in the best manner it can, just as the building produced heat. Because of the basic nature of disease, the Defense Mechanism, like the building, cannot eliminate it with the means naturally available to it. All it can do is create symptoms as a reaction to the disease's continued presence.

In the building, it is easy to see how the compensatory events or "symptoms" are an appropriate response to the cause. Even later, when the compensations extended beyond the heating system, it is still easy to see how they came about. As bad as these compensations or "symptoms" are, they did seem to make sense in this situation.

By just being aware of the reactions or compensations that occurred in the building, it is possible to guess the initial cause. That is a credit to the logic and inner structure of the building's operation and the predictable nature and evolution of these events.

The same logical, predictable development of compensations, or symptoms, occurs in us, although this is often harder to see. The principle, however, is exactly the same. Your Defense Mechanism uses its own perfect wisdom in choosing the precise symptoms that are needed to compensate for the disease. These symptoms maintain balance or homeostasis with the least possible interference to your overall freedom and functioning. Unlike the example, the initial disease cause in a patient may not be known, only the effects or symptoms are available for evaluating the situation.

Even without knowing the cause or disease, we can

understand it by examining the symptoms. This only works if we assume that the symptoms are perfectly logical compensations by the Defense Mechanism in response to a disease. If, on the other hand, we approach this analysis with the idea that these symptoms are merely random or that they are the "enemy" to be individually treated and suppressed, then no unifying system will be evident.

A possible reaction of the building's management company would be to ignore the initial problems. That is exactly what we do with so many initial symptoms that our Defense Mechanism creates.

We all frequently ignore the initial signals that something is wrong.

There are many reasons for this: we are often too busy, the symptoms are very minor, there is no time or money to go to the doctor, or we may lack awareness that what is happening is a genuine symptom.

By ignoring initial symptoms, more and more symptoms occur, often affecting areas seemingly unrelated to those presenting the initial problem. This is similar to the situation in the building as other areas and departments began to feel the unpleasant results of the continued presence of the broken window. This spread of symptoms to other areas is often what convinces doctors and patients, that they are suffering from several different diseases, rather than many aspects and consequences of a single disease process.

Without any intervention, the disease and the resulting progressive display of symptoms and problems will continue to get worse over time. When persisting symptoms concern us, we will go to the doctor for medical assistance. Conventional medical care typically evaluates only the physical body and then each medical specialist only concentrates on his own area.

There are some rare practitioners who have a broader perspective and realize that the mind, emotions and life of the person are all intimately involved in a patient's health. Yet when it comes to treatment, even they use an approach that is almost exclusively physical and symptom oriented. Medications are administered to alter, suppress, eliminate or modify single symptoms. In the vast majority of cases of chronic disease, daily medications are required to control symptoms.

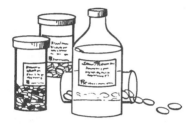

Doctors frequently treat only the patient's isolated symptoms. Patients, too, with their demands for immediate and symptomatic relief, perpetuate this type of treatment. A rash appears and an ointment is applied, the blood pressure goes up and an anti-hypertensive medication is given, a headache starts and a pain medication is used. There are thousands of examples showing this symptom oriented approach to disease. The body, in its wisdom, created the symptom through the Defense Mechanism as a natural response to the disease situation. The doctor then gives medicine to take away that very symptom. The two are working at cross purposes!

We all know that there are great advantages in taking care of problems properly from the very beginning. In many areas of our lives, we do this automatically. How strange that we often forget to do this in the most important area of our lives, our own health. It's certainly not because we don't want to take care of ourselves. We just don't realize that our present actions are not helping. Doctors dispense and people take medications with the mistaken idea that they are, indeed, curing the cause of the problem.

The whole philosophy and perspective of our medical system today is designed for immediate symptomatic relief; naturally we assume that is the correct approach. Despite being treated by the latest medical knowledge and technology and although the majority of people have adopted this form of treatment, illnesses are increasing in severity and continuing unabated.

Being unaware
of the damage and consequences
of symptomatic treatment
does not protect us from the
inevitable, harmful results of that treatment.

A less obvious but even more damaging effect of symptomatic relief through taking conventional drugs is their long term effect on our immune system, an important part of our Defense Mechanism. With this kind of treatment, the immune system doesn't have the chance to develop, to be active and to work in its normal way.

The immune system, like other organ systems such as the muscles, bones, lungs, heart and digestive system, needs to be used to stay in top running condition. Imagine what would have happened to your leg muscles if you had never been allowed to walk. Your heart and lungs increase in efficiency and health when they are used to their fullest extent as when performing aerobic exercise. Much attention is given to the importance of allowing these and other organ systems the opportunity to function in their normal way. It follows then, that the immune system also needs the opportunity to function and stay proficient at what it is designed to do.

Instead of allowing the Defense Mechanism and immune system the chance to fight off disease by themselves, we continually give "assistance" in the form of medications. We take almost every opportunity to prevent them from working. For example, by taking antibiotics to treat even the simplest infection, our immune system is not called into action and is not used for its intended purpose - eliminating infection.

This is similar to a child learning to use the dictionary. Imagine your child seated at the kitchen table writing a paper for his class the next day. He thinks of a word that he would like to use but doesn't know how to spell. Naturally, he asks you. You can make it easy for him by simply spelling the word, or you can insist that he look it up in the dictionary. If you make him look it up, you are going to get objections! "How can I look a word up in the dictionary if I don't know how to spell it?"

It is a lot more work for you to guide him in the use of the dictionary, listen to the arguments, and contend with his resistance, than simply to tell him how to spell the word. Why then do you still insist on subjecting your child to the ordeal of learning how to use the dictionary?

You insist because you know that telling him how to spell a specific word now prevents him from developing the skills necessary to spell words for himself in the future. You would be depriving him of the opportunity to learn something for himself and he would be avoiding the struggle that is a necessary part of this learning process. The path of least resistance now would cause greater difficulty in the future. Your effort to "help" him would hinder him by perpetuating his dependency on others for assistance in spelling unfamiliar words. Your child would be weakened with a limitation of his freedom.

A subject mastered results in greater freedom.

If the immune system is being continually deprived of the opportunity to function because it doesn't get challenges or "exercise", then it too will develop weaknesses, become incompetent and will eventually malfunction.

Many believe that today's destructive diseases involving the immune system are a direct result of the frequent and long term use of medications that interfere with the proper development and functioning of the immune system.

The rapid and devastating appearance of AIDS has brought a great deal of attention to the immune system and what happens when it is not working correctly. There are other diseases too, which are also known to involve a problem in the immune system. These include multiple sclerosis, rheumatoid arthritis, lupus erythematosis, certain kidney and thyroid diseases, and a whole class of diseases called auto-immune in which the immune system attacks the body's own tissues and destroys them.

Serious infections or other diseases should not go untreated. Homeopathy is very successful at treating them, including the childhood illnesses that are now subject to immunization.

There is a group of people, including physicians, who believe that having illnesses like measles, chicken pox and mumps is actually of great benefit to a child's immune system. It is thought that immunizations preventing these diseases deprive the child's immune system of the opportunity to fight them. This hinders the immune system from developing its proper strength and may have a long term adverse effect on its ability to function properly throughout life.

The immune system, like every other system in the body, has a very precise, systematic way of growing and developing. Certain aspects of the immune system must be formed at certain times. Once this time has passed, there is never another opportunity. Let's look at another part of the physical body to explain this idea. A child has a very definite pattern of development. Holding his head up, talking and feeding himself all must occur at specific ages otherwise there is something wrong. He also must walk at a certain age. There is a time in the child's development when his brain, nervous system, bones and muscles are all coordinated and mature enough to begin walking. His body weight is also just right for his muscles to have enough strength to stand and take those first steps. Walking enables his leg muscles to become stronger at the same time that his body grows, requiring more strength in the legs to support it. If that precise time passes and he doesn't begin to walk, then the growing child becomes too heavy for his unexercised muscles to support him and he can't walk. As he continues to grow, there is even less chance that he will walk. The critical moment has passed and the body's perfect system of development has been interrupted.

Immunizations also disrupt natural development. Without exposure to childhood illnesses allowing the immune system to work, it is likely that critical aspects of the immune system's development are being interrupted. These could very well result in weaknesses and handicaps in our immune system from which we never recover.

Fortunately, it is not necessary to subject children to the full effects of these childhood diseases for them to benefit fully from the illnesses's effects on their immune system. Each of these diseases can be successfully treated by Homeopathy which spares children a large part of the suffering while improving their immune system at the same time. Remember Thomas from chapter one!

Questioning the beneficial effects of immunizations is considered heresy. This is especially true when presenting these ideas to those older parents who remember the devastation or the deaths that often resulted from the diseases that have now been all but eliminated. It is presumed that these diseases were eliminated by immunizations. Epidemiological evidence shows, however, that many were already in decline before the widespread use of immunizations.

Our medical "victory" through immunizations is clouded by the fact that we now have the other devastating diseases mentioned above that cause far more suffering than these childhood diseases. One conventional medical report from the Institute of Medicine supports these ideas. Researchers found that childhood immunizations may result in episodes of inconsolable crying in infants, acute arthritis, loss of consciousness and other problems. If immunizations are linked to the modern increase in chronic diseases, this should be determined as soon as possible. Obviously, more investigations and research need to be done into the entire question of immunizations.

What we have learned so far supports this idea that there is a link between immunizations and chronic disease. Let's use the graph from chapter eight that shows the levels of Defense Mechanism functioning and specific symptoms.

Measles, mumps, chicken pox and other childhood illnesses each "reside" at a certain level on the graph. A child needs to be at this specific level of Defense Mechanism functioning to have these symptoms. We know there are only two ways to eliminate a symptom. You must either go up or down the graph. Either the Defense Mechanism gets stronger or gets weaker. To avoid a childhood disease, the child must have a stronger or weaker Defense Mechanism than is required to develop that disease.

Immunizations work by weakening the Defense Mechanism. The child is now too sick, too low on the graph, to develop those symptoms. A disease is still active in him and will present itself through more serious symptoms later. It may not even be that much later. Many parents are well aware of an immediate decline in their child's health after immunizations. The disease process started by the immunizations continues to develop. This explains why chronic disease or symptoms of a more serious nature can be linked to immunizations. These long term effects have not been fully appreciated or considered.

How is treatment with Homeopathy beneficial when antibiotics or immunizations are so harmful? Allowing the symptoms of the disease to develop and then treating with the proper Homeopathic remedy helps the body by strengthening the entire Defense Mechanism, including the immune system. The symptoms go away because the person goes "up" the graph.

Fortunately for our survival, our Defense Mechanism and immune system can withstand many interfering elements. It often takes many years, with or without conventional treatment, before the deterioration in the Defense Mechanism's functioning will become evident as symptoms. This great length of time between the interfering factors, such as immunizations or medications, and the development of symptoms makes it less likely that we will make a connection between the two events.

Homeopathic medicine and treatment provide an alternative and most often a better way to treat disease and obtain true health. Now that you have a greater understanding of these comprehensive ideas about health and disease, it is possible for you to make more informed decisions about your life and the type of medical care that is right for you.

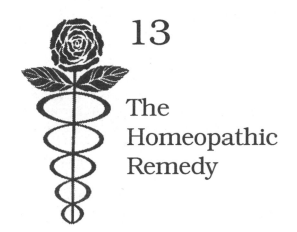

13

The Homeopathic Remedy

I have mentioned Homeopathic remedies frequently throughout this book and have included some basic facts about them. Let's look at them more closely. They are derived from plant, mineral and a few animal substances and processed in a unique manner that removes any toxic properties while enhancing their medicinal and therapeutic effects far beyond that of the original substance.

The unique preparation of these natural substances which turns them into Homeopathic remedies is one of the three key elements of Homeopathic Medicine and probably the least understood. The other two key elements, the use of one remedy at a time and prescribing for a patient according to the Law of Similars were discussed earlier.

The essence of Homeopathy's unique processing technique is quite simple. It's so simple in fact, that anyone can prepare a remedy for themselves, just as many early Homeopaths did.

This processing technique is another of Hahnemann's great discoveries. Many substances which were needed and could be used as medicines were, themselves, very poisonous.

To use them safely, it was necessary for Hahnemann to reduce the dose. He continuously learned about the healing effects of many substances in a variety of dosages. Because of his meticulous observations and experiments, he discovered something that has been an enigma to physicians, scientists and patients since the introduction of Homeopathy nearly 200 years ago. Hahnemann discovered that, oddly enough, the more dilute a substance was made, the more powerful the healing effect became. This may seem to contradict common sense and logic, yet it is none the less true.

The processing technique involves a series of dilutions of the original substance. Between each dilution, the vial containing the substance is pounded vigorously on a firm surface. This pounding is called succussion. The alternation between dilution and then succussion further increases the medicinal effects, eventually producing the Homeopathic remedy. The picture below explains this process even further.

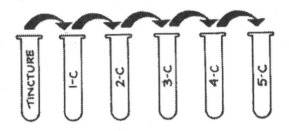

The vial on the far left contains the leaf of a plant mixed in water. This is the herb or tincture preparation of the plant. The first dilution is one drop of the original solution put into a new vial that contains 100 drops of water. The vial is then succussed. The next dilution is one drop of this solution put into another vial with 100 drops of water and this is then succussed again. This process continues.

Homeopathic remedies are labeled with a letter indicating the amount of dilution during each step and a number showing how many times that is done. A dilution ratio of one drop into ten, 1/10, is labeled "X", and one drop put into one hundred as in our example, 1/100, is "C". When this is done once, it is called 1 C, twice is 2 C and so forth.

Chemically, there is a limit to the number of times a substance can be diluted until there are no molecules left in the solution. This limit is reached when the serial dilution just described is done 12 times, or 12 C. This may seem inadequate, but actually, the amount of dilution that occurs after 12 steps using the serial method is the same as putting a single drop of the original substance in a volume of water equivalent to Lake Superior!

Homeopathic remedies commonly used are much more dilute than 12 C. They are either 30 C, 200 C and frequently 1000 C, 10,000 C or even 50,000 C!

This aspect of Homeopathy does not seem logical when viewed from the current model of science. There is, however, a logic, order and consistent behavior to these preparations that indicates science and principles are involved in their action. To understand this part of Homeopathy we must view a wider perspective of the physical world and science. Just as Newton couldn't have imagined that time could be variable, so too, we must consider a world different from our current model to understand how Homeopathic remedies are prepared and work in the human being.

How is it that these remedies still have action at these extraordinary dilutions? There couldn't possibly be any effect from the chemicals in the original substance because there aren't any molecules left. Yet, the remedies still produce a therapeutic action. How are these dilutions, which we call remedies, different from pure water? Someone once described Homeopathic remedies by saying "if a little is good, then nothing is better!" How can we be certain that there is nothing in the remedies when there are observable and measurable results in the people who take them?

There is currently a theory that explains how the processing technique of dilution and succussion could produce a powerful healing medicine from a natural substance. We know that preparation of a remedy by dilution only, without the succussion steps, results in an inactive solution. Therefore, succussion provides a vital link in the complete activation of the Homeopathic remedy.

What happens to the solution during the act of succussion? How does this pounding change the solution from one that is therapeutically inactive to one that is powerfully effective? Is there a special ingredient that is the active part of the original substance. The tremendous dilution by water of the original substance points to water as being very important in this process, possibly carrying or transmitting this active healing ingredient. Another reason that water is uniquely qualified to transfer the active agent of healing through many dilution steps is its particular and special chemical feature. Water is a di-polar molecule.

This special attribute of water can be explained with the assistance of the illustrations below. The first diagram shows the chemical structures of the components of water, hydrogen and oxygen.

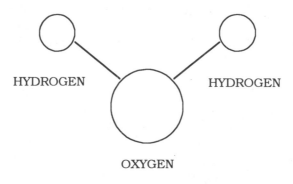

HYDROGEN   HYDROGEN

OXYGEN

Chemically, the levels or rings around the nucleus of an atom represent energy levels. An atom is most stable when an energy ring is holding its full capacity of electrons. The first ring requires two electrons to complete its energy capacity while the second ring requires eight electrons. Elements vary in the number of electrons in each ring, generally filling the inner most ring first.

Since it only has one electron, hydrogen requires only the first ring or level. Oxygen, however, has eight electrons, two in the first ring and six in the second ring. The hydrogen atom must give up its electron or get one more to make the first energy ring stable. Oxygen would be more stable with a full eight electrons in the outer ring. This tendency to fill or stabilize their outer rings causes the hydrogen and oxygen atoms to bond together in a mutual sharing of electrons. Oxygen "accepts" and hydrogen "gives" the electrons.

Since oxygen requires two additional electrons, it bonds with the single electron from each of two separate hydrogen atoms thus completing its outer ring. Each hydrogen atom will share an electron to "empty" its ring, thereby making its ring more stable. The chemical bonds between the oxygen and the hydrogen hold the molecule together. We can see this in the following diagram.

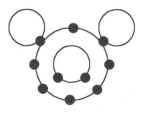

WATER MOLECULE
WITH ELECTRONS

These bonds are not symmetric. The oxygen with its larger nucleus and greater number of electrons in its outer ring has more "pull" on the shared electron than does the hydrogen. The shared electron will be drawn closer to the oxygen side of the bond than to the hydrogen side. This uneven pulling results in more of the negative charge of a shared electron being on one side of the bond and less on the other side. This is known as a di-polar bond. Despite its greater force on the shared electron, the oxygen does not have the power to pull it off the hydrogen completely. It can only cause the bond to be asymmetric or di-polar.

Nature, hardly an idle force, will not allow negative or positive charges to stand around by themselves, they always attract each other. The positive side of the uneven di-polar bond from one water molecule will be attracted to the negative side of the di-polar bond of another water molecule. This process of attraction involves all the water molecules and continues until a lattice network forms.

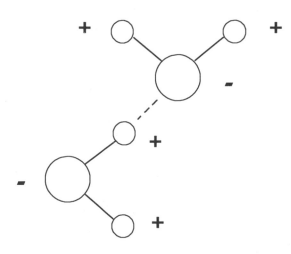

Each substance in nature has a unique and distinctive chemical structure composed of atoms and molecules, with many positive and negative charged particles. Of course, this is true of the plant and mineral substances used for Homeopathic remedies.

A specified amount of water is added to the initial substance. The positive and negative charges in these substances attract and interact with the positive and negative sides of the di-polar bonds in the water molecules. This creates a precise lattice framework. The original solution or tincture therefore contains the initial medicinal substance, surrounded by its own unique water lattice, determined by its chemical structure. Its identity is encoded in the lattice. This lattice would remind you of lace or a net with a characteristic design woven in it.

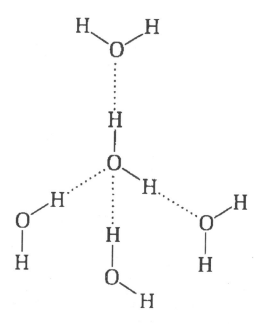

The next step, succussion or vigorous shaking, is essential to activate the Homeopathic remedy. The force of the succussion breaks the lattice into smaller pieces, each carrying the identity of the original substance through the pattern of its bonds. As more water is added for the next dilution stage, it interacts with the pre-existing lattice fragments to rebuild the lattice networks. This process is similar to taking "cuttings" from a plant. The cuttings then develop into plants which are identical to the original. As the succussion and dilution steps continue, the lattice is continually broken into pieces and then rebuilt by the addition of more water.

There is no doubt that all the original chemical substance is removed from the preparation very soon after the dilution and succussion processing begins. Information about the substance, including its medicinal properties, remains and is transferred to the solution of water by an "energy imprint" in the bonds of the specific lattice formation. Homeopathy uses the medicinal effects of the original substance through the therapeutic action of these information carrying energy bonds.

The medicinal properties of this energy bonding system in the lattice are always present and available in every substance, including conventional medicines. Due to the presence of the chemical substance in these medications, the effect of the energy in the bonds of the lattice is too weak to be felt. The chemicals overpower this energy.

By removing the original chemical in the Homeopathic remedies, we allow the therapeutic action of the more subtle energy aspects of the substance to be seen without being overshadowed by the effects of the chemical substances. This dilution also guarantees the complete safety of Homeopathic remedies. There is no chemical substance remaining to cause adverse reactions such as allergies, side effects or interactions with other chemicals.

This theory about the possible mechanism for the action of Homeopathic remedies answers many questions. Yet, there is currently little demonstrable scientific evidence to support it.

Whatever it is in the remedy that is acting to cure people, it cannot yet be measured by current technology.

That is hardly a discredit to Homeopathy. Historically, there are many examples of currently "visible" and measurable aspects of the physical world that were beyond measurement just a short time ago.

> *"All things are possible*
> *until they are proven impossible*
> *and even the impossible*
> *may only be so, as of now."*
> *- Pearl Buck*

There was a time when we were certain that there was nothing inside an atom and that it was the smallest indivisible particle of matter. Though the Greeks of the 5th century first proposed the atom theory, it was generally ignored until the early 1800's when the Englishman John Dalton demonstrated the existence of atoms in different elements and their predictable behavior in forming compounds. Nearly a hundred years passed before the atom lost its place as the most basic, indivisible and fundamental component of matter. There was just no way to detect smaller components. In 1897, the electron, one of the particles that makes up the atom, was discovered by Joseph Thompson. Other atomic components, neutrons and protons, were later revealed by others. In the minds of scientists, these particles had replaced the atom as the most basic building blocks of matter. This idea did not last long.

In 1932, the same year the neutron was discovered, a sub-particle related to the electron, called the positron, was found. The detection of dozens of additional sub-particles that are either components of electrons, neutrons and protons or related to them soon followed. If this isn't mysterious enough, since 1964 physicists have believed something even smaller, the quark, is the most elemental particle of all.

These and other scientific discoveries were made possible by two very independent factors, both of which are crucial to the advancement of knowledge. The first is the improvement in technology that allowed detection of things previously unmeasurable. For physicists, this meant machines, like the particle accelerator, that allow indirect observation of these particles and the visualization of their actions.

These and other machines have made enormous contributions to science and have been essential for the verification of previously unobservable phenomena and theories about the nature of the physical world. As soon as scientists accepted one explanation of the elemental and fundamental ingredients of matter, advancing technology provided new information which necessitated a revision of those theories and ideas. All areas of science, including medicine, are subject to this dynamic aspect of discovery provided by the explosion of technological expertise.

Radio is another good ex-
ample of this phenomena. Two
hundred years ago, we had no
idea of the tremendous amount
of electromagnetic energy or
other waves that exist in the
environment. They were always there, but not detectable
until a machine, the radio, was
developed that could translate
this energy into a form that we
could recognize; sound.

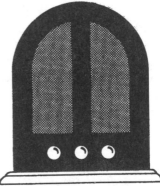

We are still waiting for a machine that can detect and translate the active energy in Homeopathic remedies into a form that we can recognize. This certainly doesn't mean that this energy is not there!

The second factor important to most discoveries is the

curiosity of the investigator. Although a many great things have been discovered seemingly by accident, the majority have been a result of the receptive, inquiring and creative minds of the researchers themselves. In the 1930's, the existence of the positron and other elemental particles was only theoretical, having been predicted by the quantum theory. These intangible possibilities and ideas aroused curiosity and the search for them began.

Technology follows the needs of scientific research itself. The desire to verify what theory and observation suggest results in the need for instruments and machines to assist these endeavors. The particle accelerator came into existence as the knowledge of sub-atomic particles grew. Once there was curiosity to learn more about these particles, the instruments to accomplish this were invented and perfected. Once bacteria and the world of micro-organisms were discovered and linked to disease, there was an interest in better microscopes. Galileo and his use of the telescope opened a whole new area of science. Continued improvement of the telescope was needed to answer the probing questions of later astronomers. The same principle applies in most aspects of science.

Technology also follows thought. Technology advances only in those areas of inquiry that are open to the inquisitive and probing minds of scientists. If any aspect of nature, science or the world is dismissed, then no technology will be forthcoming to help provide that very essential, demonstrable supporting evidence. The pre-existence of scientific evidence is often the criteria that science uses to decide whether something is worth studying. Yet this very criteria limits the possibility of obtaining the necessary collaborating data in legitimate areas of science that may be new or based on independent observation. This closes the door to development of the kinds of technology required to provide the scientific support needed. This circuitous spiral of limitations accounts for the presence of unexplained, yet observable phenomena in science, and especially in medicine.

Homeopathy and its remedies are a perfect modern day example of this bias. The remedies can demonstrate their profound action on people, yet few investigations have been made, or machines devised to measure their active aspect. The presupposition that they cannot possibly be active is the very obstacle that precludes the development of the technology which would verify the action of Homeopathic remedies to the satisfaction of the scientific community.

Physicists also encounter perplexing and unexplained events in their own field that have defied current logical thought. For example, some of the active elementary particles of matter have no mass. They are not composed of anything that can be weighed! For most of us non-physicists, it is perplexing how these particles, the building blocks of matter, can lack the fundamental requirement of all matter: measurable weight. Physicists now confirm that all matter is energy. The quantum or wave theory of matter is the foundation for this idea. Reaching beyond the boundaries of conventional thought, this innovative theory regards the physical world in terms of waves, particles and energy. It states that there are no actual electrons as isolated physical units. They and all other particles of the atom are simply energy moving in certain localities in space! Furthermore, other theories state the more you try to measure these things, the less likely you are to obtain any reliable results!

Historically, the science of biology has been at least 100 years behind physics. What the physicists discover becomes widely known and accepted relatively quickly. When applied to the human being, however, these same laws are very slow to be accepted. In practical, real terms, medical science just does not accept, believe or understand the idea that the human being is energy and is more than a physical, material body. Energy applications to medicine and the human being are still primitive at best and usually rejected or ridiculed. Somehow the human being is the only exception to these universal principles of energy and matter that physicists have developed, tested and proved.

There is a philosophy that states, "Homeopathy can't possibly work, therefore it doesn't work." A better statement would be, "Homeopathy works, therefore how does it work". If current logic or scientific methods alone say it can't work, then it is necessary for researchers to do what true investigators have always done: explore new possibilities with creative and innovative approaches to explain how Homeopaths worldwide get their remarkable results.

Homeopathy provides
a unique opportunity for
new discoveries and understanding.

Our discussion of the biological and physical laws involved in the preparation and action of Homeopathic remedies demonstrates their consistency with other aspects of nature. Relying on the advanced concepts that twentieth century physicists have contributed to our understanding of the world gives Homeopathy an even more secure place in the framework of modern science.

Years to come will build on these preliminary areas of research and the theories applying this knowledge to medicine. More sensitive instruments will detect the electron bonds, lattice work of water, the force fields and energies in the Homeopathic remedies. The future is very promising for more discovery about the potential for using energy in the healing arts. In the mean time, while this technology is being developed, Homeopathy and its remedies still work reliably to cure patients.

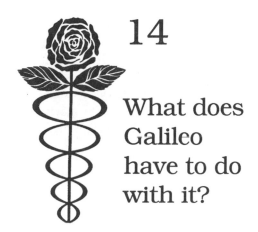

14

What does Galileo have to do with it?

Most people first hear about Homeopathy in bits and pieces: a magazine article, a film clip on the morning news or an advertisement in the local pharmacy. They might even hear about it for the first time while sitting next to me on an airplane! These fragments sound amazing and too good to be true. Most people's initial reactions to Homeopathy range from enthusiasm to guarded curiosity to down right skepticism. As with many ideas and traditions in our culture, the very fact that Homeopathy has been around for so long gives the impression that there must be some truth to it. Homeopathy would otherwise have long since disappeared as just another system that couldn't stand the test of time.

My medical colleagues, scientists, patients and others often challenge me to address their skepticism about the effectiveness of Homeopathy. I really like skeptics! It's very important for us to be discerning and questioning. It's a mistake to accept anything blindly and I wouldn't want anyone to accept Homeopathy just on my word alone. I certainly didn't accept it until I had made a thorough investigation and demanded to be shown ample evidence for the ideas and claims that Homeopathy makes.

Although I encourage you to be skeptical and critically evaluate all the evidence, you will also need to have an open mind. There are rewards for being receptive to all new possibilities. Great and significant discoveries have been made because the investigators had unbiased attitudes, and were willing to acknowledge whatever results their search produced. The impartial yet discriminating mind has the highest possibility of finding the truth.

I was greatly impressed by my initial exposure to Homeopathy. But before I could accept ideas that challenged conventional medical science as I knew it, I needed more compelling evidence to support my initial impression. I was inspired to inquire, investigate and find out for myself whether or not the claims and philosophy of Homeopathy were true.

What I discovered was quite amazing. I saw a medical system that was based on order, principles and natural law. I also witnessed incredible things happening with patients. Disease conditions that I had been taught were incurable, chronic and unrelentingly progressive were being improved dramatically or even cured. My reading, studying and classes provided considerable evidence from video cases, patients, other medical doctors and historic documents to demonstrate and verify the claims of Homeopathy. The more I investigated and learned from the masters in the field, the more I became convinced of the effectiveness of Homeopathic Medicine.

Although the popularity of Homeopathy is rapidly growing, relatively few people have heard of it and fewer still really understand it. Much of the philosophy and many of the ideas of Homeopathy are contrary to commonly held opinions and attitudes. Fortunately, diversity of opinion is one of the great freedoms we enjoy today. Homeopaths and their patients certainly hold the minority viewpoint! Just because someone has a minority opinion doesn't mean he is wrong. Galileo is a case in point.

Galileo was born in Italy in 1564 during the time of Europe's emergence from the primitive and repressed feudal life of the Middle Ages. Those centuries of repression had all but extinguished the light of philosophy, inquiry, reason and curiosity. In that era, the Church was extremely powerful, controlling every aspect of people's lives: their jobs, marriages, places of residence, clothing and even their thoughts. Even royalty had little ability to ignore the dictates of the Church. From our vantage point, it is difficult even to imagine what absolute power the Church had over the people.

Scientific inquiry, as we know it, did not exist. The Church's interpretations of the scriptures was absolute, dictating the philosophical and moral context in which the people lived. Without freedom to question Church doctrines, no advancement of knowledge was possible.

Among the Church's teachings was the idea that the Earth was the center of the Universe. Although man was created in God's image, he was only rarely considered divine. He was usually thought of as a lowly sinner, fallen from grace in the Garden of Eden. Despite his tarnished and flawed nature, man and therefore his home, the Earth, was still considered the center of the Universe because of his Divine connection.

The first person who openly questioned the Earth as the center of the Universe was an amateur astronomer named Copernicus who did his work before the birth of Galileo. Copernicus, a physician and church canon, was an active leader of his diocese. Though astronomy was only a hobby, he devised an entirely new system of positions of the heavenly bodies. He proposed that the Sun, not the Earth, was the center of the Universe. Furthermore, he stated that all the other planets, including the Earth, revolved around the Sun. His ideas were founded and developed on a theoretical basis, deriving information from the classic texts in geometry, philosophy, astronomy and mathematics. Copernicus knew that his ideas of a sun-centered universe lacked actual collaborating evidence and violated the contemporary thought of the day, including the Church dictates. He, therefore, chose not to publish his ideas during his lifetime. They were first released in 1543, at the time of his death.

It was Galileo who provided the first observable evidence to support the ideas that Copernicus had developed from theory. It was the discovery and use of the telescope that brought the visions of the heavens to Earth and with then came a turmoil of change.

In the early 1600's, news of the telescope was spreading slowly through Italy. It's invention, most widely attributed to Galileo, was actually the work of a Dutch spectacle maker. When the Senate of the city-state of Venice decided to purchase such as instrument for maritime and navigational purposes, it was a long time friend of Galileo who was in charge of the project. Galileo, an inventor and instrument maker in his own right, was given information about the telescope so that he might make a better one for the Senate. The commission came in the summer of 1609 and by the end of that year, Galileo had perfected and improved the telescope beyond that of previous instruments. He had turned this "toy for seeing at a distance" into the instrument responsible for the eventual adoption of a Sun-centered universe.

Then Galileo turned his telescope skywards and was awe struck by what he saw.

Initially, Galileo and his telescope were applauded. Theologians, mathematicians, Church leaders and even Pope Paul V honored his discoveries. This favorable and open reception was short lived. Almost immediately, the more prevalent conservative members of the Church began to investigate Galileo and his teachings.

There was enormous resistance by these members among the church leaders and established community to even look through the telescope themselves which, they argued, deceived the God-given senses. They would not trust information from an instrument over their direct first-hand experience with the naked eye.

Galileo's first accounts of his telescopic voyages to the heavens (1610) caused great alarm and consternation among his peers. The real trouble began, however, with his report of seeing Jupiter and its previously undiscovered moons. This meant the Earth with its moon was no longer unique. Additionally, measurements of the moons' motions around Jupiter confirmed a planetary system in which the Sun was the center and the Earth, like Jupiter, revolved around it.   Prior to his investigations, Galileo had supported the accepted Church doctrine of the Earth-centered Universe. The evidence provided by his telescopic discoveries changed his views.

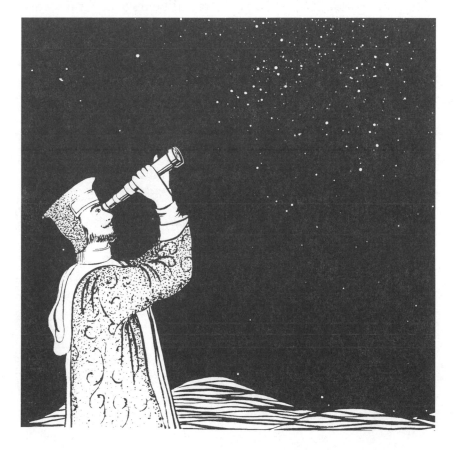

The theories of Copernicus, published over half a century earlier, finally had observable and measurable evidence to support them. Before the telescope, these ideas posed little or no threat to the established Church doctrines. Even Copernicus was somewhat well tolerated because he produced no evidence for his ideas, which therefore could be easily dismissed. Galileo was now a very big threat by actually demonstrating supportive facts that anyone could see through the telescope.

Despite being prohibited from publishing a new treatise in 1616, Galileo continued his research, writing and teaching about a Sun-centered universe. He was absolutely compelled to tell the truth of what he saw. The publication of yet another book on the subject in 1632 proved to be the last straw for the Pope. Beleaguered as the Church of Rome was from a growing Protestant faction, the Pope took this opportunity to exert his power and consolidate the authority of the Church. These political events, though unrelated to Galileo and pure science, had a profound effect on the Pope's decision to finally censor him.

During a trial in 1633 in Rome, the Pope not only completely censored the offending publication, but insisted that Galileo recant his views publicly and remain imprisoned. The written recantation is a matter of historical record. Galileo remained imprisoned for 9 years until his death at the age of 78.

Galileo put his faith in what he experienced and witnessed. He was interested in whatever his observations and Nature revealed to him. His virtually single handed efforts to contribute to a larger, more complete understanding of the world, were accompanied by the risks that come when one is presenting ideas that are contrary to prevailing thought.

He continually pursued the path of truth in spite of the overwhelming majority opinion, including scholars, citizens and theologians who were supported with power, tradition, wealth and religious commandment. His courage to do all this was fortified by the truth that he perceived.

In many ways, being a Homeopath today is similar to

Galileo's situation. His observations were absolutely contrary to the beliefs of his day. The ideas of Homeopathy are also contrary to current conventional medical thought even though these ideas have been derived from careful and accurate observation of Nature. The Church of Galileo's era was no more powerful or influential than the conventional medical establishment is today.

It is easy for us to look back at Galileo with admiration and scoff at his opponents and detractors. It is important to remember, however, that at a time of any major change in fundamental ideas, there is naturally great resistance, opposition, confrontation, and difficulty. Our natural tendency is to resist change. Today, Homeopathy is in the forefront of a dramatic change in the way we understand the human being, how disease is developed and how health is maintained. Regarding the human as a whole, integrated, functioning being with physical, emotional and mental aspects that are all interwoven and impact health is one such revolutionary change in perspective. These current changes are equal in importance and consequence to those that resulted from Galileo's discoveries.

In reading this book, you will undoubtedly encounter ideas that are new to you and may challenge the way you view the world, especially the world of health and medicine. Remember Galileo and the fact that his ideas were also new and challenging in their day. Historical perspective has exonerated Galileo. I encourage you to follow Galileo's example and evaluate the concepts in this book with an open and inquiring mind, and even with an eagerness to know the truth. Then you will have a glimpse into the new understanding of the world that is emerging around us.

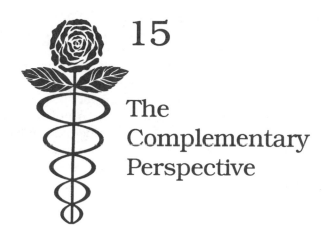

15

The Complementary Perspective

Society's growing awareness and fascination in medical care, healthy living and preventive health measures have produced an explosion of information. Our curiosity and interest naturally extend beyond the confines of commonly accepted conventional medicine toward Alternative or Complementary Medicine.

In England and other European countries, the term Complementary Medicine is used to refer to therapies outside the mainstream of modern conventional medical care. This is more appropriate than our term "Alternative Medicine" since it suggests the idea that the various forms of medicine complement and assist each other. The ability of each medical system to complete and provide what is deficient in the others sets the stage for cooperation and partnership in the shared goal of assisting a suffering humanity.   Indeed, each system has something to offer and the most appropriate one should always be used at any given time. Unfortunately, this does not often happen.

There are many types of therapy, from nutrition to reflexology, from acupuncture to massage, from meditation to kinesiology, from crystal healing to ayurvedic medicine and, of course, Homeopathy that are available and vying for consideration. Each of these and many others, are making various claims about their effectiveness and superiority. Despite any competition or disagreement among them, they are all agreed that the conventional western approach to medical care falls tragically short of doing the job of curing people. The large number of people in western cultures who are now turning to these alternative or complementary methods also reflects this realization. Dissatisfaction has grown because people are having direct experiences which challenge the effectiveness and expose the limitations of our currently dominant medical system.

The boundaries of any medical system are defined by what it can and cannot do to care for ailing people. The limits which make up the boundaries are defined by the level of knowledge, scientific advancements, the understanding of human health and disease processes as well as the attitudes, philosophy and values of society as a whole. Consider the following illustration.

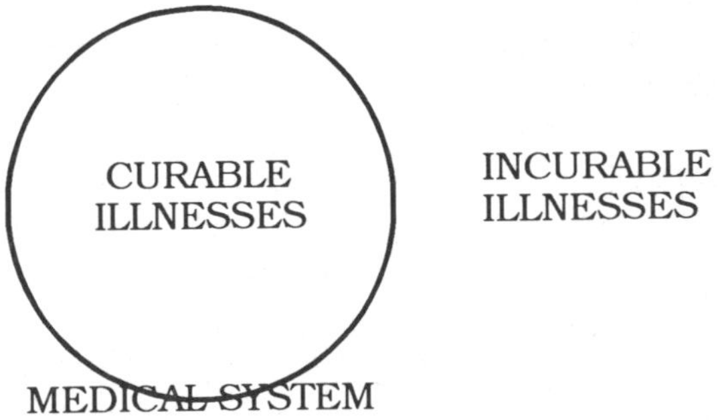

CURABLE
ILLNESSES

INCURABLE
ILLNESSES

MEDICAL SYSTEM

The circle represents western medical philosophy, ideas, methods and perspectives on health and illness. Briefly, this view regards illness as a malfunction within the body, usually unexplained, but whose immediate cause is chemical, cellular, biologic, or infectious. Therapy is aimed at this biologic, mechanistic malfunction. External intervention is needed to correct "Nature gone wrong". Furthermore, the mind and body are separate, neither having much to do with the other. The great variety of knowledge, technology and other miraculous advances are all based on the above ideas.

Inside the circle are all the illnesses and events that are consistent with this view. Any "disease" that can be cured with this medical approach is located inside the circle. As long as a person has an ailment that falls inside the circle's boundaries, no deficiency or limitation to the system's perspectives, views or therapeutics will be evident.

The world, however, is much larger than the boundaries of the current medical model. As is repeatedly and painfully demonstrated, there are many "diseases" currently not being cured by using that model and its therapies. This indicates these "diseases" must be located outside the circle.

Can the circle be expanded to include more diseases and provide for their effective treatment? The answer is a resounding YES. This is the stated objective of our conventional medical leaders, researchers and physicians. Unfortunately, the circle can't be enlarged by technology alone. Only a change in the underlying perspective, premises and principles of a medical system will cause the boundaries to expand.

Perspective, not technique, enlarges the circle.

This is a rather radical statement which many people would contest. After all, there have been many technologies that have created improvements in health. Antibiotics, immunizations, modern surgical techniques, pharmaceuticals and many other advances certainly must have expanded the boundaries of that circle. Each has, indeed, changed medicine and our health in dramatic ways. Each, however, was preceded by and developed from a change in perspective, attitudes and philosophy about human beings.

*We cannot solve a problem with
the same way of thinking
that created the problem.*

The discovery of antibiotics is a perfect example. For all practical purposes, the age of antibiotics began in the 1940's with the "discovery" of Penicillin. The action of Penicillin was actually first noted in the middle 1800's. It was observed that the mold, now known to produce the chemical Penicillin, stopped the growth of other kinds of "growing substances". They didn't know about germs or bacteria yet, so this observation didn't mean anything. It had no meaning or value until after Pasteur, Koch, Lister and others in the late 1800's confirmed the existence of bacteria and implicated them in disease. Once bacteria or "growing substances" were thought to be the cause of disease, then the observation that there were molds that could stop their growth had an entirely different significance.

The idea that bacteria exist and that they cause disease is a change in perspective which altered the foundation premises of medical thought. Only then were the techniques for eliminating bacteria developed.   The use of antibiotics is only one technique that resulted from these new views.   Hygiene and other sanitation measures to reduce contamination from disease-producing bacteria played a major role in the reduction of illness and deaths during the years between the "discovery" of micro-organisms in the late 1800's and the development of antibiotics in 1940.   Modern surgery also hinges on these perspectives; it is possible only in a bacteria free environment.

There is a dynamic quality to the nature of ideas and perspectives as new discoveries change attitudes, thoughts and concepts. One example is the growing realization that our minds may actually be involved, somehow, in the functioning of our bodies. This new view provides a broader perspective than that previously held. This simple, yet dramatic change in the fundamental premise from one in which the mind and body are disconnected to one in which there is a relationship between them immediately enlarges the world view and consequently enlarges the circle. There are many for whom these ideas seem obvious; they have already changed their perspective.

When the perspective changes and the circle enlarges, therapies whose worth were previously questioned are then taken out of the closet, dusted off and given a fresh look.

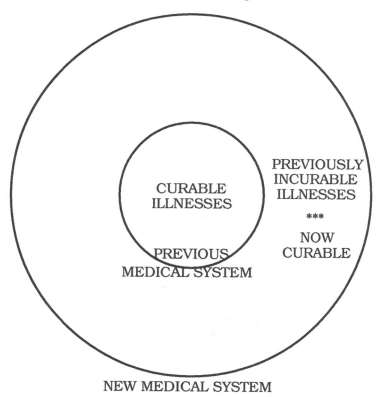

NEW MEDICAL SYSTEM

Such disciplines as biofeedback, hypnosis, and stress reduction are gaining new interest. Their effectiveness in helping
many conditions that were "resistant" to conventional treatment have further added to their prestige and acceptance. In
addition, most have received the final accolade: they are paid
for by medical insurance companies.

Additional medical conditions that were previously outside
the circle's boundaries and therefore considered "incurable"
are now inside its borders. They are now treatable because they
are included in the expanded circle. The specific techniques
themselves, such as biofeedback or hypnosis, are less important than the appearance of the idea itself. Once an idea is
thought to be true, then all kinds of techniques inevitably
follow.

*The foundation (idea) must be there before
the structure (therapy) can be built upon it.*

There is a fascinating story which exemplifies this concept.
Norman Cousins's book *Anatomy of an Illness* details his
personal story of health, medicine and changing perspectives.

On the very first page of *Anatomy of an Illness*, Mr. Cousins
states "People wrote to me to ask if I had 'laughed' my way out
of a crippling disease that doctors believed to be irreversible".
This opening statement alone gives a clear indication that there
is a different perspective being used here! Reading on we find
other statements such as "I had a fast growing conviction that
a hospital is no place for a person who is seriously ill". This
confirms that Norman Cousins does not have the same world
view as the majority of the medical profession.

Norman Cousins's experience began in 1964 when he was
suddenly and mysteriously afflicted with an unusual disease.
It began as a mild aching in his bones and quickly progressed
to increasing pain in most of his body and joints, accompanied

by extreme exhaustion. His condition was so serious, he had to be hospitalized. Faced with the diagnosis of chronic and incurable "collagen vascular disease," Cousins began to research the cause and cure for his terrible malady. Having been in the vanguard of current literature and medical thought for many years, he reread the books that addressed issues of stress and its impact on health. He reviewed the events which had happened just before the onset of his illness and found several emotionally and physically exhausting and stressful events. Without too much surprise, he related them to his current condition.

Cousins's recovery began when he asked this question, "If negative emotions produce damaging chemical changes in the body, wouldn't positive emotions produce healing chemical changes in the body?" He wondered if love, faith, and laughter would have therapeutic value. With the support and cooperation of his physician, Cousins set about developing a plan to put his ideas into action. He devised a complete "regeneration" program to help his body in its efforts to heal. Whereas love and faith were immensely important, even more so was plain old fashioned laughter. The pragmatic side of Cousins nature wanted a systematic approach. He began watching funny movies and television clips and discovered that ten minutes of laughing would relieve his pain for up to two hours!

The combination of his newly discovered "laughter therapy" and large doses of Vitamin C resulted in his gradual improvement for the first time since the onset of the disease. He was soon able to leave the hospital and eventually regained the use of his joints and extremities. Complete recovery took many months, but any recovery at all was well outside the predicted outcome for this "disease" through conventional medical treatment.

Both Norman Cousins and his remarkable physician adopted a whole new perspective when evaluating and treating this illness. Cousins applied his scholar's mind to the problem, evaluating and researching his own situation in a logical and thoughtful way. Cousins hadn't simply "laughed" his way out of a life threatening illness, he demonstrated that the full range of positive emotions, combined with a logical, scientific approach to illness can yield dramatic results. The mistaken idea that any treatment or theory of disease that is outside the realm of conventional medicine is lacking in logic, analytical thinking and reason is challenged by Cousins's careful approach and account of his experience.

When Cousins saw the limited choices available from within the circle of the conventional medical world, he immediately expanded that circle for himself. His perspective of the human being as an integrated whole, which is affected in significant and important ways by the emotions, stress and nutrition, allowed a broad and inclusive enough therapeutic approach that literally saved his life.

The circle that now represents Norman Cousins's world view of medicine, health and healing is defined by his own poignant statements taken from *Anatomy of an Illness*: "It is possible that these limits will recede when we respect more fully the natural drive of the human mind and body toward perfectibility and regeneration. Protecting and cherishing that natural drive may well represent the finest exercise of human freedom."

As Norman Cousins's story so dramatically illustrates, it is possible to expand the circle representing conventional modern medicine. This will include as many illnesses as possible inside the new border to help as many people as possible. It does require fundamental changes in the accepted perspectives, philosophy and views of the world. How can we go about doing just that? The first step is a commitment to examine, question and evaluate the philosophy and premises, indeed, the very foundations of the current medical system.

It is often difficult for us to examine our own premises because we regard them as truths. If something is true, why question it? As truth, how could it possibly be changed?

*We feel so strongly
that our beliefs and premises are true
that every aspect of our whole life,
including our medical system,
is built on and around them.*

Premises, however, are not truths, they are just ideas that
we think are true. With life orchestrated around these premises, we continually reinforce, confirm and verify the "truth-
fulness" of these glorified opinions. Our medical system is built
on these premises that define what will be regarded as illness,
what will be accepted as appropriate therapy and the extent to
which the system will be willing to change itself. Because the
majority of people share these same premises, this has helped
solidify the current system and fortify its doctrines against
question, challenges and, of course, against any change.

The first time we suspect that one of the "truths" in the
foundation of our view of life is not solid is when we have an
experience that defies this "truth". When events occur that do
not fit into our currently held world view, we "bump up" against
the boundary of our personal circle.

John Enright Ph.D., a brilliant and innovative psycholo-
gist, wrote and taught extensively about premises, how they are
formed, how they are used and how they limit us on all levels,
as people, families, societies and nations. He coined the term
"premise shock" to describe the unsettling, but liberating,
experience of discovering that the foundation on which we
stand and depend is actually the shifting sands of expanding
awareness. Each of us goes through this process - if we are
lucky. The result of experiencing "premise shock" is the
expansion of our perspective and the enlargement of our
personal "circle", leading to a larger, fuller life with a greater
experience of freedom, creativity and happiness.

Dr. Enright's choice of the word "shock" in "premise shock" is highly significant! There can be great discomfort when a firmly held truth, the glue that holds everything together in our life, is no longer regarded as an inviolate and undeniable fact. Often we must restructure our life after one of these experiences. Consequently, these realizations are often stubbornly resisted and avoided.

To avoid these realizations, we restrict ourselves to those events, people, thoughts and actions which pose no challenge or threat to our existing premises. We must live within the boundary established by the currently held premises. Graphically, we will stay within the circle, avoiding anything that happens to fall outside.

This enormous reduction
in freedom and choice in our lives
is the price we must pay for
holding on to an outmoded opinion
as if it were "truth".

Disease is also a reduction in our freedom; resisting the changes that follow a premise shock can cause and maintain an illness.

Although, premises and the experience of "premise shock" are fairly common and occur to many people, they are often not identified as such. Here is a case in point.

Until the turn of this century, the world view of physics and Natural Law was dominated by Newtonian thought. Sir Isaac Newton's explanation and model of the world were taken as a truth. His reasoning and descriptions of nature were impeccable. The Newtonian view put systematic order and logic in the universe, providing explanations for phenomena that were previously observed but not understood. The elegance, beauty and harmony of his ideas were unsurpassed and stayed that way from the time Newton began his work in 1660 until the beginning of the 1900's.

Then in 1903 the world underwent a "premise shock". Einstein published his work on relativity with the matter-energy equation. This challenged all our assumptions about how the universe worked, how it was made and by what rules it operated. The Universe, presumably, had not changed. What had happened, was that Einstein found a circumstance in which the premises that had been operating no longer worked. He stepped outside the circle. Once this happened, it was clear that what had been thought of as absolute truth, was only "the truth" under certain circumstances. Now a new, expanded version of truth had to be developed, one that applied to both the new and the old situations.

Newtonian physics assumed that time was constant and unchanging. Certainly that is very logical and indeed it is true, but only in environments which are well below the speed of light. Einstein discovered that as the speed of light is approached, time becomes variable. Newtonian physics, lacks provisions to account for the fluctuations of time as this circumstance was not anticipated. This theory, therefore, is no longer adequate to explain phenomena which are observed at speeds approaching the speed of light.

Newton's set of formulae, definitions and his assumption that time was unchanging define the boundary of the circle. Einstein's work explained and redefined the boundary.

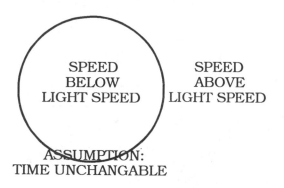

SPEED BELOW LIGHT SPEED

SPEED ABOVE LIGHT SPEED

ASSUMPTION: TIME UNCHANGABLE

Those events occurring well below the speed of light where time is constant will be located inside circle. Those events occurring near the speed of light will show a variable time influence and will not fit Newton's formulae or framework. These events, therefore, occur outside the circle.

Any boundary or limitation is invisible until an event that doesn't fit bumps up against it. Einstein's great achievements include the fact that he found such an event. Even more remarkable is that he did not dismiss his observations and ideas because they were contrary to ideas and mathematical formulae that had been held as absolute truth for 300 years and a world view that had been in existence since - well, the beginning of *time!*

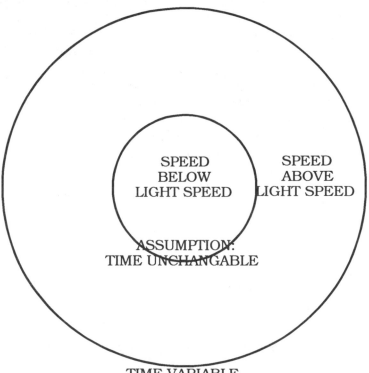

SPEED BELOW LIGHT SPEED

SPEED ABOVE LIGHT SPEED

ASSUMPTION: TIME UNCHANGABLE

TIME VARIABLE

Einstein's new premises, perspectives and resulting formulae, provide an expanded, more comprehensive view of the universe. He expanded the circle so more conditions and circumstances of life are now located inside that newly defined circle.

Einstein did not negate Newtonian physics. He began with Newton's concepts and expanded them. Any expansion of the circle always includes all that the circle contained before and then adds more to it. It is truly an expansion, not a replacement. Newtonian physics is still applicable in our everyday lives, because very few of us need to consider events that take place when approaching the speed of light. None the less, we always benefit, directly or indirectly, from an expanded, more complete perspective of the world.

Medicine is currently going through a "premise shock". The old tried and true perspectives, methods and premises of the conventional medical system are being challenged in ways that are impossible to ignore.

There are increasing numbers of events and circumstances that cannot be explained using the established ideas.

Growing public interest in alternative or complementary forms of therapy also shows that there are increasing numbers of people whose premises and world views are changing and becoming fundamentally different from those of modern medicine. As a medical consumer, you are growing more independent and demanding change or expansion of the boundaries of conventional medicine.

Medicine as a system now has the same opportunity that we do when faced with experiences that defy our world view and concepts. It can and should expand and change its perspective to a broader, more comprehensive view by seriously evaluating and examining those events and episodes that challenge the existing order.

So far, the medical system and some of the people who comprise it, have seemingly closed their minds and ignored the existence of events that are not explained by the current medical model. Norman Cousins's physician proves that there are individual doctors who are open-minded, curious and innovative. There are many open minded, progressive people in all branches of the medical profession. Unfortunately, their impact on the fundamental structure, opinions, and methods within conventional medicine is still limited. Only by changing can medicine effectively respond to the needs of the very people it hopes to help.

One reason for the difficulty that the conventional medical world has in accepting Homeopathy is that the two systems are based on entirely different world views. As long as the conventional world retains the premises and medical model it now holds, it is unlikely that its practitioners will begin to understand how Homeopathy works, or even that it does work. It is frustrating to Homeopathic physicians to show evidence of cured patients to a conventional medical doctor, only to have the cases summarily dismissed.

The view from the vantage point of Homeopathy (the expanded boundary on the circle) encompasses both the previous circle's content and the new area. The view from inside the original boundary, however, cannot see the expanded one. Homeopaths can see the premises and understand the world view of the conventional medical doctors but those doctors often cannot comprehend the ideas of the Homeopaths.

This is similar to a person with perfect color vision trying to explain color to someone who is color blind. The world views, literally and figuratively, are very different. They are located on different boundaries of the expanding circle: black and white sight, the limited view, is located on the inner rim and full spectrum sight, a more complete view of the world, is represented by the outer border.

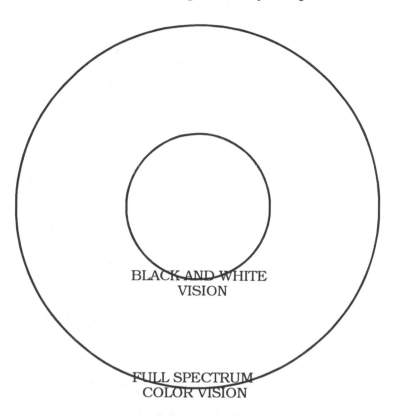

BLACK AND WHITE
VISION

FULL SPECTRUM
COLOR VISION

The full spectrum sighted person also can see black and white, but this is not so for the black and white sighted person. He cannot see color. How could those who are color sighted tell the others about color? What proof, research studies, documented evidence could possibly convince the black and white sighted that this thing called "color" really exists? None of the evidence would have any effect at instructing about color since it would all be seen in black and white! This is similar to watching a color movie on a black and white television set. Since color is not in their range of experience, it is unlikely that the black and white sighted people will change their opinion.

What is needed is a fundamental change in their visual

apparatus to enable them to see color and therefore move to the outer rim of the circle. If this could occur, then this new world "view" would immediately lend credence to everything that the full spectrum sighted people had said all along.

*A change in perspective
is the only "evidence" needed.*

As long as conventional medical philosophy remains unchanged, it is unlikely that the doctors and other professionals in it, will accept Homeopathy. Any evidence that is produced by the Homeopathic world to prove its validity will always be evaluated from within the boundary of the conventional medical model. This is similar to black and white sighted people evaluating from their perspective the evidence that demonstrates color.

The circle, now defined by conventional medical thought and philosophy, will be greatly expanded by adopting the larger world view which serves as the foundation principles of Homeopathy. These Homeopathic premises, philosophy and ideas will not negate any of the current knowledge. They will expand what is known and provide the ability to operate from a more comprehensive perspective.

When more medical conditions are located inside the circle and are within the therapeutic reach of an expanded medical system, it will be possible to provide greater assistance to a troubled world. This is the gift that Homeopathic Medicine offers.

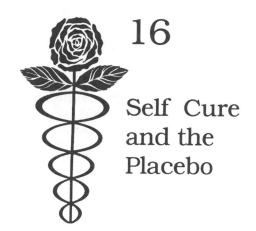

16

Self Cure and the Placebo

The effect of our minds and attitudes on illness and disease is an area of human physiology and psychology receiving increasing amounts of attention. We are now taught that the mind can do many things to overcome illness. A patient who wants to get well, who has a positive attitude and who does biofeedback, imagery and affirmations can reduce or eliminate symptoms. This can help him cope with a disease and minimize its effects on his life.

These methods are often just not enough to remove the disease and its symptoms completely. Homeopaths often treat people who have already done or who are doing many different self-help activities. Besides using the power of the mind and a positive attitude to overcome illness, many have tried nutrition, exercise, meditation, herbs, vitamins and other therapies. Often, however, they cannot find the complete relief they are seeking. If they could have activated their internal power for self-healing, they would be well by now.

*The inability to achieve a self-cure is
a very important symptom.*

Often the disease involves our mind and emotional areas. This blocks our normal ability to generate healing emotions and positive mental states that can produce beneficial changes in us. Trying to cure ourselves by using the same areas that are affected by disease is often impossible. It would be like trying to lift yourself three inches off the floor by the scruff of your neck!

The disease also can block our ability even to begin the process of inner healing. Our inability or lack of desire to do those things that we already know are good for us constitutes a very significant set of symptoms. Homeopathy is effective in breaking though the disease-generated barriers so the mind can resume its normal contribution to our cure.

There are many instances when the disease process interfers with the ability of the sick person to do what he needs to do to improve his health. For example, someone who craves sugar knows that he feels much better when he doesn't eat it, yet frequently the desire for sugar overpowers his will to resist. The sugar craving is a symptom of the disease process, which interferes with the desire to maintain optimum health. Similarly, someone who doesn't exercise may feel too tired to do so. He feels better after he exercises, but fatigue prevents him from doing it consistently. The fatigue is a symptom of a disease process that interferes with the ability to do exactly what would bring him relief.

*The inability to make the changes
that would contribute to our health is
a significant symptom
and indicates the presence of disease.*

The dramatic and miraculous improvements seen after Homeopathic treatment result from elimination of the disease which created symptoms that inhibited the natural inner drive toward health, balance and freedom. This is shown frequently by cures in people who have tried many other methods for self-healing, including the power of their own minds in addition to conventional treatments.

For the person with sugar cravings, Homeopathic treatment removes the disease which causes that symptom, thereby making it easier for him to eat in a healthy way. For the person who lacks the ambition to exercise, this symptom, too, will be improved once the Homeopathic remedy has eliminated the underlying disease process.

As any Homeopath will tell you, it is easier and more enjoyable for people to do those things that are healthier for them after they have had proper Homeopathic treatment.

*As we get healthier,
we are naturally drawn to
those activities, attitudes, foods and lifestyles
that are better for us!
This is part of total health.*

Once we have been cured of disease, we also have more ability to withstand adverse conditions brought about by poor diet, a stressful or sedentary lifestyle and other problems or potential disease influences.

Though we better tolerate a poor diet when we are healthier, we just don't want to eat that way. Cravings for sugar, junk food, salt or snacks can disappear altogether. We want healthier foods! All this occurs naturally, without effort or forced dietary restriction. The entire gastrointestinal tract becomes healthier and functions better. Food eaten gets digested, used and stored in a far more efficient and appropriate way. The result is a normalization of the appetite and eating patterns. Other people find themselves wanting to exercise, whereas before treatment they were always too tired or just couldn't seem to find the time. The normalization of all the systems of the body brings an overall state of good health. When that happens, the patient experiences many delightful and unexpected surprises.

Some skeptics say that Homeopathic remedies are just placebos, inactive substances or "sugar pills" being used as medicines. Homeopaths are often accused of "talking" their patients into better psychological states and then giving them a remedy that lacks any real effect. They say that the placebo effect is the only possible explanation for the disappearance of symptoms and improvement in the patient's health after a Homeopathic remedy. A remedy is definitely not a placebo. I sometimes wish I had the power to cure people by placebo. It would be so much easier than the precise, rigorous and often extremely difficult Homeopathic medical system.

The suggestion that Homeopathic remedies have no effect other than what the patient creates for himself based on a placebo effect is totally unfounded. There is a wealth of evidence and clinical experience supporting our claims of much greater effects from Homeopathic treatment than that of placebo.

There are several groups of patients who respond very well to Homeopathic treatment in whom a placebo effect is unlikely, if not impossible. These groups are animals, infants and young children, the unconscious and even people who doubt that Homeopathy really works.

The Law of Similars works even when patients are not aware of it or do not believe in it. This is very much like having an x-ray exam. The x-ray machine produces a picture even if the patient does not believe it's possible. The repeated and consistent results from the x-ray machine have made everyone confident that it will work even if they don't know exactly how it works. No one says that it won't work simply because they don't completely understand it.

Although many may not completely understand or accept Homeopathy, it will still cure them.

There is a unique quality about Homeopathic treatment that verifies its activity and separates it from placebo. This characteristic is known as the Homeopathic aggravation. Frequently after administration of the appropriate Homeopathic remedy there will be a slight to moderate increase in the patient's symptoms. Typically, this occurs within the first several days after taking the remedy and lasts from several hours to a week.

By looking at the Law of Similars (chapter ten) we can understand how and why this occurs. As you recall, this biologic principle states that a sick person will be cured when given a medication that is known to produce those same symptoms in a healthy person. The patient is receiving just that much more ability to produce the very symptoms he requires to eliminate his disease.

After receiving the correct Homeopathic remedy, the Defense Mechanism produces the symptoms it needs in a more intense way because it now has enough power to rid the body of the disease. This period of intensification of symptoms signifies healing activity, showing that the remedy has acted. Then the disease is eliminated and the symptoms improve.

This period of aggravation never occurs when a person is treated with a placebo. For decades, researchers have used placebo in a variety of investigations without ever showing this intensification of symptoms.

Patients who really want Homeopathy to work for them would be the most likely to be affected by placebo. Their desire to get well, their belief in the effectiveness of Homeopathy and their confidence in their physician are all factors that would contribute to the placebo effect. If all improvements with

Homeopathic treatment could be attributed to placebo then these people would improve without any aggravation of symptoms. Under Homeopathic treatment, they too show an aggravation of their symptoms. Furthermore, the incorrect remedy has no effect, despite these patients' great belief in Homeopathy.

Evaluating, diagnosing and prescribing the one correct Homeopathic remedy for a patient can often be a difficult process for the doctor. He must follow the Homeopathic method in a very precise way to achieve positive results. He must perceive and record the symptoms accurately and prescribe by the Law of Similars, using the data available in the Materia Medicas. If he does not follow this method, or gives a Homeopathic remedy randomly, then there will be no result, no improvement in the patient and no improvement of the symptoms.

Only the one correct remedy works to cure; the other remedies will not work.

If the results of Homeopathic treatment were all due to placebo effect, then all this time and effort would not be needed. Belief in Homeopathy by the patient would be enough.

Once the Homeopath prescribes a remedy, both the doctor and the patient believe the correct remedy has been given. If this remedy gives no change in the health, the doctor will prescribe a different remedy. When the correct remedy is given, there will be an improvement. A placebo would have shown a similar result for both remedies.

Placebo does not have the predictability of Homeopathic treatment. Response to placebo occurs randomly and depends on the patient, the physician and the circumstances. Research studies evaluating the effects of placebo, report a 30 - 40% overall response rate. On the other hand, highly skilled Homeopathic physicians often show a highly predictable 90% positive response rate.

Homeopathy is the third largest system of medicine in the world. It is second largest outside China where acupuncture is used extensively. In France alone, there are about 12,000 medical doctors who practice Homeopathy either full or part time. There are 100,000 in India and many thousands across Europe, South America and Mexico. England has several dozen schools for training Homeopaths. Other European countries, including Germany, Holland, Belgium, Scotland and Sweden also having training programs. The British Royal family uses Homeopathy and has a private Homeopathic physician. In several European countries only fully licensed medical doctors may prescribe and treat patients with Homeopathy.

These doctors are highly trained professionals and many have attended the same medical schools as their conventional counterparts. Is it possible they cannot tell the difference between the results of a placebo and that of Homeopathy? Are all these physicians giving placebos in the name of medical science?   If so, why are their results so much better than research studies using placebo?

If the thousands of documented Homeopathic cures of multiple sclerosis, ulcers, hypertension, depression, eczema, asthma, infections, ulcerative colitis, migraine headaches, ovarian cysts, fibroids, prementral syndrome, panic attacks, hepatitis, Epstein Barr virus syndrome, herpes and so many other problems were helped simply by placebo, then why isn't placebo used more often? If placebo is so powerful, why isn't the conventional medical community using it to cure patients with less effort, expense and fewer side effects?

The answer is that Homeopathy cures according to biologic and scientific law and not by placebo effect. This is far more consistent with an ordered, predictable, harmonious world based on Natural Law.

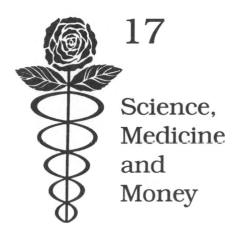

17

Science, Medicine and Money

Patients come to Homeopathy because they have seen it work for others and stay because it works for them. Doctors become Homeopaths because they witness over and over that it works.

The scientific research and investigation that is usually done in conventional medicine has had very little to do with Homeopathy's popularity, use by medical doctors or its widespread acceptance by people who have chosen it as their preferred medical system. In previous generations, Homeopathy gained fame because of the dramatic and remarkable results it achieved during the frequent epidemics of that time. Malaria, cholera, typhus, and scarlet fever were all treated very successfully by using remedies, saving countless numbers of lives.

There is currently a demand for Homeopathy to meet the rigorous scrutiny of the scientific method that other treatments and therapeutics must go through to gain official approval and acceptance. This would demonstrate to the conventional medical world, in a form it respects, that Homeopathy is both effective and free from adverse effects.

There has been very little interest by Homeopaths in doing the kind of research that is usually done in medicine and science. It simply isn't needed. For their knowledge, Homeopaths have relied mostly on observation of disease, treatments, the action of the remedies as well as their experience of treating patients. There are thousands of documented cured cases that cannot be explained on any other basis except that Homeopathy truly works. Those scientific investigations and publications that Homeopaths have been doing for over 150 years are generally limited to the provings of remedies and other clinically useful information. Homeopaths have also published individual case reports, and information about specific remedies. For all practical purposes, no other research has been done.

The scientific method has been developed over many years to eliminate the uncertainty and unreliability of using an individual doctor's observations and experience or single case reports. Modern science organizes and objectively evaluates the validity of data from observations and theories. The demand now is to subject Homeopathy to this type of evaluation rather than allow its acceptance to be based on pre-scientific assessment, case reports and doctors' individual experiences.

There is very little modern research and few published investigations which demonstrate the claims of Homeopathic medicine. It is generally assumed that this is because the claims can't be proven. This is definitely not so. To illustrate, I will briefly describe three recent major studies published in the conventional medical literature.

The first, published in the Lancet, a well respected British medical journal, is a study of the effectiveness of Homeopathy in the treatment of hayfever entitled "Homeopathy - is it a placebo response?" This study showed conclusively that positive reaction to the Homeopathic remedy in the hayfever sufferers was far better than the reaction to a placebo. Despite this well controlled study and its conclusions, one skeptical doctor remarked, "They have just substituted one placebo for another!"

The second article published in the British Journal of Pharmacology detailed a study showing Homeopathy to be effective in limiting the symptoms of arthritis sufferers. There were far fewer side effects or toxicity in the group treated with Homeopathy than was experienced in the group treated in the conventional manner. The conclusion of the researchers was support for Homeopathic treatment.

The third article published in the prestigious science magazine *Nature* in June 1988, details the exciting research of Jacques Benveniste MD, a famed French researcher. His five year study shows an effect on human white blood cells after the administration of a substance prepared by the method used for Homeopathic remedies. This effect was absent when giving placebo.

Many are still skeptical of Dr. Benveniste's work and his surprising results. Yet the spirit of scientific curiosity and integrity is prevailing as several laboratories in other countries are now replicating these findings and pursuing other avenues of research along these same lines.

Having research studies to support an idea or theory is not the final accolade. Not everything that influences a human in health and disease can be tested in a research study.

Being a physician is as much an art as it is a science.

Practicing doctors and other clinicians rely on many other factors to diagnose and formulate treatment plans. Doctors draw upon their experience, observations, clinical data, empirical results, financial and legal considerations when doing their job. These factors are typically not included in research studies.

There are many problems in using a research study for evaluating the effectiveness of a particular treatment. There are many difficulties in designing any study with appropriate controls to minimize interfering factors.

The typical clinical studies done by most pharmaceutical companies, researchers and universities, are known as double blind studies. In this type of study, neither the doctor giving the medicine nor the patient taking it knows whether their dose is the drug being tested or a placebo. It is the most highly respected type of research and considered the "gold standard" in conventional medical research.

Most research studies, including double blind studies, are designed to eliminate as many variables as possible to show the effectiveness of a single medication. Individual differences in the patients being studied are standardized using a few broad categories such as age, weight, sex and race.

People, however, are not so easily categorized. We all have emotions and minds and we are influenced by hundreds of other known and unknown factors. We live in an ever changing environment that cannot be standardized or controlled. Moon phases, sun spots, meteorological factors, life events, job stresses, seasonal variations all affect us in varying degrees. Yet in the midst of this chaotic array of influences, scientists assume that research studies eliminating these very factors will yield results that are significant enough to apply to the treatment of people in their natural environment and regular life.

There are other serious if not impossible problems when attempting to use the double blind study for conducting research on Homeopathic remedies.

The problems of doing conventional research on Homeopathy are inherent in its very nature which has individualization as its key feature.

The whole idea of eliminating the distinctive features of a person's symptoms for the purpose of standardizing a research study is contrary to the very nature and principles of Homeopathic medicine.

For example, a typical double blind study would test the effectiveness of Homeopathic treatment on 100 headache sufferers. Half the patients would receive a Homeopathy remedy and the other half would receive an inactive sugar pill. This standard approach does not individualize treatment and would give all patients who received Homeopathy the same remedy. Only those few patients needing that particular remedy would respond favorably, showing dramatic improvement. The others would show no change, or some mild improvement similar to those who received the placebo. This kind of study would obviously not reveal the full potential of Homeopathic treatment.

On the other hand, if the study permitted each individual to receive his correct remedy according to the Law of Similars, then the improvement rate of these patients would be very high, well above what would be expected from placebo.

Another outstanding feature of Homeopathy is long term improvement in health.

It is common for a patient to have continued improvement for many years. Evaluating someone's overall life and health after several years of Homeopathic treatment reveals dramatic results. Most research studies, on the other hand, assess the outcome of a therapy after just a few months. Short term evaluation limits the possibility of seeing the benefits of Homeopathy for eliminating chronic disease.

Cancer research is one area where long term evaluations are common. Five and 10 year survival rates are routinely collected and studied. Homeopathy could definitely show how effective it is in curing so many devastating chronic "diseases" if its 5 and 10 year cure rates were collected. There is a great improvement with Homeopathic treatment as compared to accepted statistical progress for these same "diseases".

An additional difficulty with the double blind study is the isolation of a single symptom or "disease". Understanding Homeopathy, we know that different symptoms in different areas or organs of the body are not separate diseases, they are the same inner disease process. Testing and comparing the effectiveness of one remedy against another for curing a specific symptom has no meaning in Homeopathy and is not even possible.

With these major problems and differences, how can anyone expect Homeopathy to be tested by double blind studies? Once all the unique factors in Homeopathy are accommodated in the research study, there is very little left of the standard double blind study.

Compare this to a master chef hired to prepare his specialty, a delicious cake. The chef's reputation relies on the result and satisfaction of the guest, a visiting dignitary. Naturally, he wants to do his best. Before beginning, the chef is informed that the guest is on a diet, therefore, he can't use sugar. The guest also has an allergy to eggs, cannot digest flour, has a milk and cream intolerance and won't eat butter because he is trying to lower his cholesterol. Despite these problems, the chef is still required to prepare his special cake and maintain his reputation.

This is exactly what is expected of Homeopathy. By using the double blind research method, standardizing the factors, evaluating only one symptom, short term follow up and lack of a holistic perspective, no favorable result could possibly occur. They would be taking away all the ingredients that make Homeopathy what it is and would still be expecting results! I invite the conventional medical doctors to meet Homeopathy's standards of cure which demand improvement of the whole person.

There is still an emphasis on the double blind study as the means required to convince the conventional medical community of the validity of Homeopathy. This is especially interesting since there are other areas in medicine where the double blind study can't be done. Cancer, transplantation, surgical procedures and psychiatric therapies all have special research requirements to demonstrate their effectiveness.

It is possible to do research on Homeopathy, however, a new approach to research design, purpose and goals is needed to incorporate Homeopathy's unique features.

Research studies must allow Homeopathy
to reveal all it can do and
verify all it has done
for patients for the last two centuries.

Here is an example of a well designed study for Homeopathy using childhood ear infections. We have three different children, each with an elevated temperature and a bright red bulging ear drum that is extremely painful. All conventional doctors and Homeopaths would agree that each child has an inflammation of the middle ear.

So far only three symptoms, elevated temperature, ear pain and bulging ear drum, are incorporated in the diagnosis and treatment plan. Now let's look at the additional individual symptoms. The first child is crying softly, clinging to its mother and quite shy with the doctor. In spite of his painful ear, he allows the doctor to use the otoscope to examine it. The child sheds a few more tears and tries to hide in his mothers arms. The second child is crying very loudly. His aren't the only ears that are hurting - everyone else suffers too! This child is angry, irritable and will not let the doctor even come near him. He is inconsolable and ill-tempered. Nothing pleases him! He always wants to be carried by the mother but even this doesn't satisfy him. The third child is listless and sleepy with a bright red, flushed face and a very high fever. His symptoms came on very suddenly. This is usually the child whose parents call for an emergency appointment because of the rapid onset of the symptoms.

Although each child has an ear inflammation, we observe dramatic differences by looking at all the symptoms and characteristics from the whole child. If these children were treated conventionally, they would each receive antibiotics for up to 10 days. To a Homeopath, each child has a different disease and would get a different remedy. The first child would get a dose of Pulsatilla, the second, Chamomilla and the last child, Belladonna. In a matter of hours and certainly by the next day, each child's problem would have resolved, usually with no further treatment required for that episode.

Homeopaths have reported thousands of these clinical case reports about cured patients in published articles in Homeopathic scientific and clinical journals. The American Institute of Homeopathy has continuously published case studies, articles and other reports since it was established in 1844. The Institute was the first national medical association, preceding the American Medical Association by several years. In their demands for published evidence, the detractors of Homeopathy don't consider Homeopathic medical publications as valid. Refusal to accept this evidence eliminates the very kind of clinical documentation that is demanded of Homeopathy.

If research is required just to prove that Homeopathy, as a science or therapeutic system, is legitimate; to whom must this be proven? If the great amount of evidence, cured cases and the worldwide popularity of Homeopathy has not brought Homeopathy to its rightful place in medicine, is it realistic to think that this will be accomplished by double blind studies?

There are many factors involved in the area of scientific research that have an impact on whether research is begun and how it is interpreted. Let's put this whole issue of research into its real political, economic and clinical context. It is not now, nor has it ever been the case, that merit is the only criteria for acceptance of ideas. Power, money and politics always play their roles.

Perhaps the most important influence determining which research is done is the financial aspect. As a multi-billion dollar industry, pharmaceutical and other biomedical companies have a tremendous impact on medicine in general, and research in particular. There is always the consideration of who will pay for the research and who will benefit financially from it. When one drug is shown to be better than that of a competitor, there is a huge profit in it for the manufacturer. Fame, prestige, promotions and tenure are other advantages that come to those involved in a product endorsed by research.

There are many clear cases of vested interests in the outcome of research projects.

Because of the expense of most research done today, funding for a project is a major concern. Universities, pharmaceutical companies, and others with something to gain from a study's favorable results are often the ones who also fund the project. In recent years the whole issue of independent basic science research, product development and profit has clouded the university research setting.

Research studies and investigations should definitely not be stopped. I am only suggesting that our current methods are not always objective or reliable at face value. Alternative ways to evaluate the effectiveness, safety, and reliability of a particular treatment should be found.

It would be a great improvement to eliminate financial considerations from the research area. Those who have a vested interest in the outcome of a study should never be involved in it in any way. The complex, interwoven mesh of financial, economic and political factors in medicine and research, makes this almost impossible to do. It is, on the other hand, one of the most important areas for correction.

The situation in Homeopathy is quite different. There isn't any financial conflict between different Homeopathic remedies because all Homeopathic pharmaceutical companies make all the remedies. Research is more objective because no research is done for one specific remedy or for the benefit of one company over another. This allows for a unified interest in better understanding the human being in both health and disease, and in promoting Homeopathy as a science and method of therapeutics.

Without this profit incentive, however, it is less likely there will be funding for research projects in Homeopathy. This is a primary reason that so little research has been done.   Our system demands Federal Drug Administration approval for every drug that is marketed, a process averaging more than 7 years and 15 million dollars to complete. No wonder pharmaceutical companies insist on having a patent for each drug tested.

This economic issue points to another difference between conventional medicine and Homeopathy.

Homeopathic remedies are natural substances that cannot be patented and are incredibly inexpensive to make.

No one company can have exclusive rights for any remedy. This may seem like good news for patients, when in fact, this "advantage" is one reason Homeopathy has been opposed and suppressed by pharmaceutical companies and the conventional medical profession for over one hundred years. When a few dollars worth of Homeopathic remedy can *cure* a patient who would otherwise need $50-$100 worth of medicine each month, it does look like there might be a financial interest in discrediting Homeopathy.

There are limits to the scientific method of data gathering and evaluation.   It often excludes anything which is not consistent with its own parameters. Only accepting the double blind and other modern scientific methods is similar to only accepting information written in English. A great deal of value is neglected. This is also similar to testing a deaf person's intelligence when the only acceptable criteria is how well he can hear.

There are many examples in the history of science where valuable and brilliant discoveries came from direct observations. The nature of basic science is that an idea or observation comes first and it is then evaluated in light of the existing theories. If the new idea falls outside those accepted theories then a new hypothesis is formed to explain the observation. Experiments are then designed to evaluate the new hypothesis.

New ideas demand that experiments adjust to the requirements of the discovery. Copernicus, Galileo, Harvey, Einstein and many others developed an idea so new that different ways of experimenting and viewing the world had to be found to accommodate their observations and discoveries. This is the same process of expanding the boundaries of the circle we discussed in chapter fifteen.

Homeopathy, too, has new hypotheses, principles, and ideas based on observations. In addition, it isn't the only medical discovery that has been widely resisted despite ample proof of its effectiveness.

Dr. Ignac Semmelweis (1818 - 1865) and his discoveries provide an excellent case in point. He was a physician working in the Vienna Maternity hospital in 1846. In the hospital, there was a 10 - 30% death rate from puerperal or "childbed" fever in the women whose babies were delivered by medical students, but only a 3% mortality rate in the mothers whose babies were delivered by midwives in places other than the hospital. The situation had become so bad that women pleaded not to be taken to the hospital. The hospital's medical faculty and attending physicians had many different theories about why this discrepancy existed, among which were the weather conditions in Vienna, the mothers' anxiety about delivering or their embarrassment when being examined by medical students from other countries. While these explanations appear silly to

226 * Everyday Miracles

us, they were actually proposed by the eminent physicians of that day.

In 1847, a medical colleague of Semmelweis cut himself while doing an autopsy. The wound caused a very severe illness that proved to be fatal. Dr. Semmelweis observed that the symptoms his friend developed were very similar to those in the women who became ill and died after childbirth.

Semmelweis then discovered that the medical students in the hospitals went from working in the morgue straight up to the delivery ward. He concluded that there must be something about the morgue that contributed to the puerperal fever.

He made this observation at a time when the discovery of bacteria and the germ theory of disease were still several decades in the future. It is, therefore, even more amazing that Semmelweis insisted that the medical students wash their hands between their work in the morgue and attending patients or delivering babies. Just by adopting this simple procedure, the death rate in the hospital dropped dramatically.

We naturally assume that this simple, yet life saving discovery was applauded and supported by the medical community of that time. Actually, Semmelweis and his insistence on hand washing was met with fierce opposition, especially from his colleagues. Dr. Semmelweis's sincere conviction, based on clinical and observable results, was met with scorn and rejection. He was ridiculed for ideas that seem common place and all too obvious to us today.

Since germs and bacteria were unknown, his ideas about cleanliness and hand washing as well as his observations and experiences made no "sense" because they didn't fit into the current ideas of the day. Instead of acknowledging the dramatic results they produced, his ideas were summarily dismissed because he could not explain why his ideas worked. They didn't become acceptable until years later after the germ theory of disease was developed through the pioneering work of Pasteur, Koch, Lister and others. There was then a context that explained why hand washing reduced the death rate in the hospitalized women.

This is very similar to what Homeopathy faces today. Homeopathy can empirically demonstrate cures and improvements in health. There is clinical and observable data waiting for the scientific context to catch up. Is this vast amount of experience and help to patients going to be ignored until this happens? Will our society and medical community follow the example of Dr. Semmelweis's colleagues who let women die of sepsis while they argued about theory?

All this happened a long time ago, so we might think that nothing like this could occur today.

*Even today, valuable new ideas
are not always embraced.*

New ideas aren't accepted even when they are supported by overwhelming scientific evidence of the sort that the medical profession claims it requires. A modern day example is Henry Heimlich, M.D. He developed the Heimlich Maneuver which is used to save the lives of choking and drowning victims. Thousands owe their lives to this simple yet effective emergency treatment.

For those of us who are familiar with the Heimlich Maneuver, it may seem as if it has always been accepted. It is taught in schools and hospitals and required for primary health care providers. Its widespread use seems a good indicator of its acceptance.

That may be the case now but Dr. Heimlich had to struggle for many years to get his well documented ideas and the Heimlich Maneuver accepted by the general medical community. His is another fascinating story in the history of medicine, the nature of new ideas and the resistance to them.

Before Dr. Heimlich's work, Americans were taught that in cases of choking, drowning or for any foreign substance lodged in the throat, the victim should be firmly slapped on the back.

In 1974, Dr. Heimlich published a paper reviewing 1134 cases of choking and drowning in which back slaps either made the patient worse, or contributed to his death. This evidence was further supported by another 6000 cases from published papers dating back to 1854. All of these served to verify Heimlich's assertion that back slaps actually made matters worse by driving the obstructing object deeper into the lungs. Based on these findings, he devised the Heimlich Maneuver to expel the object or water from the lungs thereby providing relief.

His work relied upon double blind studies and research from the leading clinics and laboratories in the nation. There were also legal cases which supported his conclusions and recommended the use of the Heimlich Maneuver instead of back slaps. In these cases, juries made awards to victims who had received back slaps resulting in a worsening of their conditions. They found that these injuries could have been avoided by using the Heimlich Maneuver.

Despite this overwhelming evidence presented in the form required by the conventional medical world, the Heimlich Maneuver was not accepted by the principle medical associations of the United States.

Several states passed laws in the mid 1980's, to accept the Heimlich Maneuver. This was a direct result of the publicity of the legal cases and a ground swell of public support. It was not a result of the support from the medical profession itself or from the publication of research and double blind studies.

In 1985, Surgeon General C. Everett Koop, M.D. issued a US public health service report in which he stated that "back slaps are hazardous and even lethal." This clear, unequivocal warning was still not enough to overcome all the resistance to the Heimlich Maneuver in the medical community and some of its prestigious organizations.

Finally in 1988, fourteen years after its introduction, some medical organizations involved in emergency instruction began instructing the Heimlich Maneuver and stopped teaching the dangerous back slaps . They did not, however, warn those millions of people they had previously taught of the dangers of back slaps. Those instructed before the 1985-1988 period still do back slaps. Those groups that were so resistant to making this change never admitted their earlier mistakes.

For Dr. Heimlich, the years of struggle against political, medical and economic systems as well as peoples' personal biases have not come to an end. How many additional lives were lost is difficult to say. This modern example shows that the problems faced by Semmelweis have not gone away.

*The often repeated human tendency
of resistance to new ideas
once again plays its part in
the history of medicine and mankind.*

Homeopaths are assured that if they just had double blind studies, and scientific evidence, Homeopathy would be readily accepted by the mainstream medical world. Yet Dr. Heimlich, a respected surgeon with an abundance of just that kind of scientific evidence, has struggled for years and continues to struggle to prevent needless deaths.

Consistency and reliability are two features that are important for any medical system. Can we be sure that a treatment, medication or therapy, today, will provide long term effectiveness and safety.

*The recommendations
in conventional medicine and research
often change from year to year.*

These changing recommendations are regarded as the positive impact of progress and the medical profession's expanding knowledge and skill. This progress has lead to a dazzling array of new treatments, procedures, technologies and medications. We are often overwhelmed at the "miracles" now possible through modern medical expertise.

Not all the changes in conventional medicine are for the better. There have been many instances in the recent past where a specific medicine or treatment is determined to be safe and effective, only to be removed from the market later because of dangerous effects in humans that did not appear in the initial research studies.

Homeopathy, on the other hand, has remained consistent since its inception nearly two hundred years ago. What a remedy did then, it still does now. There are no surprises, unexpected adverse effects or unpredictable results.

Frequently, this reliability and predictabililty is criticized, stating that by not changing over time, Homeopathy has not taken advantage of all the developments and progress in medicine. Homeopathy has not needed to change! No improvement is needed or even possible in a medical system that already has reached the goal of curing disease. Only a medical system that is *not* completely effective in providing cures needs to continue to improve and change.

For example, high blood pressure can be cured with Homeopathic treatment. Why would it be necessary to try something new, develop new anti-hypertensive medications or use a different therapy when the patient is already cured? Conventional medicine, however, generally only provides continuous medication for the control of high blood pressure. Research for new and more effective medications continues because the problem still exists in the patient. The persistent presence of the disease also requires further understanding of the problems associated with high blood pressure and their treatment.

If there is an objection to the consistent, reliable, unchanging qualities of Homeopathy, it is best met with the statement, "If it ain't broke, don't fix it!"

Today, many more people would like to have Homeopathic treatment than can be treated by the available number of qualified Homeopaths. There are just not enough trained doctors and other practitioners. This has not always been the case.

In 1900, a great many doctors practiced Homeopathy and there were over a hundred hospitals where people could receive Homeopathic care. Several dozen medical schools taught Homeopathy.

Now there are no medical schools and only a handful of Homeopathic medical doctors. One of those hospitals still exists, the Hahnemann Hospital in Philadelphia, but today you cannot be treated there with Homeopathy. Currently there are no hospitals where a patient can go and receive Homeopathic treatment.

A lost generation of Homeopaths takes a long time to replace.

What happened to reverse this early trend of support for Homeopathy and result in its near disappearance? We have already talked somewhat about economic interests and the general resistance to new ideas. Now let's look more closely at the economic factors.

Homeopathic treatment is generally far less expensive than conventional medical treatment and it is easy to understand why. The action of Homeopathy is curative, and therefore, people are released from the downward cycle of worsening symptoms which ordinarily need continuous medications, doctor visits, and treatments. Without the need for extensive blood tests, x-rays, hospitalizations, procedures, surgeries and other costly medical services, the overall cost of Homeopathic care is significantly lowered. It follows that the biomedical and pharmaceutical companies, many doctors and others involved in providing the medications and services which are no longer needed, have more than a passing interest in seeing Homeopathy discredited and abolished. This may seem a bold and even shocking accusation to make, yet history has shown this frequently to be the case.

"Patent medicine" manufacturers over 100 years ago were antagonistic to Homeopaths when they recognized the impact

Homeopathic cures were having on the sales of their elixirs and potions. Political pressure financed by interested companies was partly responsible for the passage of restrictive and suppressive laws in the United States designed to eliminate Homeopathy. Medical historian, Harris Coulter, provides a thorough and fascinating account of the history of the conflict between Homeopathy and conventional medicine over the last hundred and fifty years in his well documented book *Divided Legacy, Volume Three*. He gives startling and revealing facts about the calculated, economically and politically motivated dismantling of the Homeopathic profession in this country since the mid-1800's. Today the virtual absence of Homeopathy as an alternative medical system in the United States reveals the enormous success of those efforts.

Even those areas that are less of a threat to medical services and products are still resisted by most of the conventional medical world. Recall that the Heimlich Maneuver is a simple, easy, no cost method of saving lives. Good nutrition and preventive health measures were generally not accepted by the medical community, but became popular among the public.

When the grass roots interest grew to be
a significant economic force,
then nutrition and preventive health measures
began to receive some attention from
the conventional medical world.

Part of the reason many doctors resist incorporating nutritional counseling or education on preventive measures into their practices does not actually come from them. Both of these activities involve a considerable amount of time for which they receive very little or no payment. It is more profitable to see more patients, do more testing and other procedures than it is to educate and spend extended periods of time with patients. Why is this true? The answer is very simple. Medical insurance companies pay doctors for tests and procedures rather than for spending time with patients. As long as doctors are being well paid to do procedures and are paid very little for talking to or educating patients then that is exactly how treatment will be oriented. Homeopathy is so time-consuming that it doesn't fit into the typical doctor's practice.

Here we see how insurance companies, economics and other non-medical considerations are directly dictating the kind of medicine that is available to you. When medical insurance pays a physician more to help a person stay healthy than it does for repairing the damages from not being healthy, then we will see doctors spending the time necessary to prevent and cure disease. Homeopathy will then take a major role in medical care.

Economics also plays a part in determining whether doctors will be trained in Homeopathy and choose it for a career. The training to become a Homeopathic physician is long and difficult. My experience was that learning to become a Homeopath was just as difficult and in many ways more difficult than learning to become a medical doctor and has taken just as long. Additionally, all this extra training came after I had completed my regular medical education. In effect, I've completed medical school twice! This is what is currently demanded of any physician who wishes to become a Homeopath in the United States.

Homeopathic physicians generally earn less money than their conventional medical counterparts. If Homeopaths were paid 10% of all the money that our cured patients won't have to spend on future health care, then we would have incomes similar to our conventional colleagues! We know what medical problems and expenses we are preventing!

A physician can earn a very comfortable living as a Homeopath, but this will not approach the enormous salaries that are now commanded by most of the specialists in modern day medicine. It seems unrealistic to expect that a physician, whose typical income is over $400,000 a year, would choose to become a Homeopathic physician and earn one fifth of that.

Let's not blame the doctors. Which would you choose; a job in which you earned a moderate amount of money or one in which you were highly paid for your work? No contest, right? It should come as no surprise that doctors make this same choice.

Patients, too, have contributed to making the current medical system the way it is. From the earliest times, the system has responded to patients' demands, needs and the market forces. Our desire for immediate cures, symptomatic relief at any cost and very little personal responsibility for our own health has also had its impact. Conventional treatment can provide the quick fix that we have so often demanded. It also does not require much from the patient other than taking his medicine and paying his bills.

Because most medical expenses are taken directly out of the patients' hands through insurance, often very little connection is made between the services they want and their real cost. There is a natural tendency to want "everything done for me" without any attempt to hold down the costs because "someone else is paying the bill." Doctors also do everything possible and more, because of moral, ethical and legal considerations.

Consider a situation involving the sale of a product. The consumer can have as much of it as he wants and doesn't have to pay for it. The salesman gets to decide how much of the product the consumer buys and bills another company. The company paying the bill has no method of limiting how much the consumer buys. This is basically how the medical system in this country works!

These and many other factors have fueled the financial crisis in medical care today.

Homeopathy is the silver lining to the black cloud of financial crisis in medicine.

Whenever something becomes unrealistically expensive, alternatives are sought. When gasoline prices increased dramatically in the late 1970's, suddenly solar energy, fuel efficient cars and home insulation were on the scene. The financial crisis in medical care is also making less expensive alternative methods of becoming healthier and staying that way much more popular. Homeopathy is a perfect answer to so many problems in our financially beleaguered system of medical health care.

I have already mentioned some ways in which Homeopathy can help reduce medical costs. There are many other ways, too. They are all based on the principle of curing people so they don't require any more treatment. Healthy people naturally make a better world for all of us. In addition to helping us be healthier individually, Homeopathy can also help create a healthier medical system.

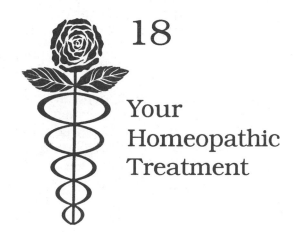

18

Your
Homeopathic
Treatment

What do you need to know before having Homeopathic treatment? Though it isn't necessary to understand Homeopathy fully for it to work for you, some information about what to expect from Homeopathic treatment will help ensure your confidence and involve you more in the healing process.

Visiting a Homeopathic doctor is usually a very positive experience. Generally, new patients are pleasantly surprised by the Homeopath's attention to all the details of their symptoms. The initial interview can last up to two hours. This is the length of time that is often necessary for the Homeopath to collect enough information about your symptoms and about you as a unique individual to prescribe the correct remedy. Only one remedy from the two thousand available will work to help you, so the Homeopath's job can be difficult.

The questions asked and the information which is useful to the Homeopath may be very different from what you are accustomed to giving to physicians. Don't be concerned if entire areas of information that are commonly needed by conventional medical doctors are ignored and entirely different areas are given great attention and concern. Remember, it is the job of the Homeopath to find the right remedy for you. He will ask only those questions that will provide the information to achieve that goal.

I have talked alot about what Homeopathy is, now you need to know what it isn't. It is not counseling, psycho-therapy, faith healing, religion, new age therapy, hypnosis, mind-over-matter or any other form of treatment where you must actively participate. The success of your Homeopathic treatment is dependant on your answering the Homeopath's questions to the best of your ability and then upon your avoiding certain substances that are known to interfere with the action of Homeopathic remedies.

You may be wondering how Homeopathy can work when it relies so fully on the patient's own story of his disease and subjective descriptions of symptoms. It is true that patients frequently can't describe their symptoms, don't accurately identify the problems involved, omit relevant details and on occasion don't even tell the truth. Even though these seem like insurmountable handicaps, methods of accommodating these considerations are built in to the system. The skilled Homeopath knows exactly how to get the information he needs. If you are perplexed by a certain line of questioning, you can be sure that your Homeopath is working diligently to identify and collect information that is of particular importance.

Frequently Homeopaths are asked to cure a "headache" or a "cold". In the conventional medical world, these complaints are generally met with an immediate prescription. For a Homeopath, it is more complex than that.

To understand these complexities better, I'll ask you to identify the song the flute is playing.

It is almost impossible for you to know which song I have in mind on the basis of the information I've given you. To identify the song accurately, you need more of the musical score.

This is exactly how it is with a "headache". Far more information about the headache and other aspects of the person is needed before the Homeopath can give the correct prescription. Just as you need many notes to identify the song, the Homeopath needs many symptoms to identify the remedy.

If there are no distinct symptoms present, the Homeopath may not identify a specific remedy. It is important to wait until the symptoms stabilize to produce a clear picture of the required remedy. The development of the disease and the response of the Defense Mechanism have a specific time when the remedy will provide the most beneficial action to you. If given too early, the remedy may not act because the Defense Mechanism may not have needed any assistance in combating the disease. Giving the remedy too late may result in an unnecessary delay for the curative action. When given at just the right time, the Homeopathic remedy provides you with the greatest benefit. This is similar to fruit ripening on a tree that must be picked at just the right moment to maximize freshness and taste.

It is very important for you as a patient, to understand this concept. You must have confidence when your Homeopath does not prescribe a remedy even though you may feel you have symptoms needing immediate treatment. The decision to wait rather than prescribe is often a difficult one and is just as therapeutic and important as taking a remedy. Too frequent administration of Homeopathic remedies or those given at the wrong time can disrupt treatment and cause progress toward good health to be delayed or reversed.

Letting your Defense Mechanism eliminate the disease by itself makes you healthier. Your entire system is strengthened when it is allowed to function on its own. Only when the Defense Mechanism cannot overcome a disease by itself does it "ask" for help by producing symptoms in very distinct, definite patterns that exactly match a specific remedy. If no such pattern appears, it means the Defense Mechanism doesn't need help yet. If your Homeopath is asking you to wait, it is because he doesn't see a remedy pattern in your symptoms and is doing exactly what your Defense Mechanism is telling him to do - wait until it calls for help.

Previous use of conventional medication usually makes Homeopathic treatment much more difficult. The Defense Mechanism has to contend with the presence of these chemicals by producing symptoms related directly to these medications. Even after stopping these medications, their effects often remain. If you have taken medication, not only are you sick from the real disease, but you are made doubly sick from the effects of the drugs. It is difficult to tell which of your symptoms and changes are from the true disease process and which are effects directly related to the drugs.

In conventional treatment, the effect on the symptoms for which a drug was prescribed is called the therapeutic effect. All the other effects of a drug are called the side effects. That is a misconception. All actions of drugs are effects, some may be desired while others are not, but they are all effects. They all impact the natural state of the Defense Mechanism and the body as a whole.

Even with an understanding of a drug's action, the Homeopath will find it challenging to understand a patient's symptom picture after it has been confused by the use of conventional medicines. A reason for this is that knowledge of the effects of conventional medications is usually limited to the physical body. Research for development of drugs and their approval for our use by the Federal Drug Administration is done mostly using animals, therefore, the effects on the more subtle and uniquely human areas of the mind and emotions often cannot be determined.

Sometimes medications will completely suppress a symptom. At other times it can change the nature of the symptoms or cause the body to produce entirely new symptoms. In all cases, the information from original pure symptoms produced by the Defense Mechanism is lost. The symptoms necessary for homeostasis are removed, altered or suppressed and the normal reactions of the Defense Mechanism are "short-circuited".

The drugs change the symptoms to such an extent that the shades of difference of their original presentation are lost, making it difficult and sometimes impossible to gather enough accurate information to prescribe the correct Homeopathic remedy. For example, there is a Homeopathic remedy which cures asthma that is aggravated at midnight. There is an entirely different remedy for asthma that is aggravated at 2 am. If the patient has been taking conventional asthma medications to stop the asthma entirely, details about the asthma are lost. Without this valuable information, finding the correct remedy can be difficult. The symptoms are the compass that a Homeopath uses to find his way to the right remedy.

If you were to take conventional medications to treat symptoms after beginning Homeopathic treatment, you could stop the action of the remedy, rendering it ineffective. How does this happen?

In chapter eight, we discussed the return of old symptoms and how that signifies that the Defense Mechanism is increasing in strength. If the old symptom is again treated by conventional medication, it will be suppressed and the disease will be driven deeper. This is the same thing that happened the first time the symptom appeared and was treated. Driving the disease deeper stops the action of the remedy.

The Homeopathic remedy increases the strength of the Defense Mechanism, conventional medications reduce its strength.

Sometimes new symptoms occur after Homeopathic treatment has begun. They facilitate the Defense Mechanism in the elimination of the disease. Symptoms frequently used in this process include skin eruptions, discharges from mucus membranes of the nose, respiratory tract, genitals and gastrointestinal tract. As annoying and distressing as these symptoms may be, it is important not to treat them. It is vital to allow your body to continue to heal in its own way and at its own pace. Any disruption by treatment to remove these symptoms, can and usually does result in the abrupt cessation of the remedy's action. There will then be a return to the declining function of the Defense Mechanism that caused all the problems in the first place.   You should always inform your Homeopath of any changes in symptoms so that he can make the proper analysis and treatment if needed.

Many diseases start because minor skin rashes were suppressed by medication.   In these cases, there is a high probability of the return of some kind of skin eruption during the course of treatment. I've explained this so frequently to patients that many of them tell me "I know you're going to be delighted--I've got a rash now!" Imagine going to a conventionally trained dermatologist and having him congratulate you for getting a skin rash!

Many patients become worried about having their old symptoms return. They often vividly recall the discomfort, pain and misery they suffered with those previous symptoms. The mere thought of having to go through that all again is frightening.

The return of old symptoms
should be a cause for happiness
because it signals that
the process of restoring good health
is underway.

Several things about the return of old symptoms need to be kept in mind. First, not all the previous symptoms will come back. You are more susceptible to the symptoms at a particular level but may not develop them during the healing phase.

Second, often the healing process is rapid, allowing the Defense Mechanism to move very quickly through a level of activity where a certain set of particularly distressing symptoms were originally produced. The speed at which the Defense Mechanism moves up through the levels is dependent on several factors: the length of time you had the major symptoms, the amount of conventional treatment you had, your total general vitality and your heredity.

Symptoms rarely come back at the same intensity and duration as the original form. During the original presentation of the symptoms, the Defense Mechanism was declining in function and the cause of the disease was still present and active. After taking the Homeopathic remedy, the disease is gone and the Defense Mechanism is regaining more power and activity. The result is a greatly reduced presentation of any returning symptoms during this healing process.

The most important thing to remember about the return of the old symptoms is that you are now moving away from ill health.

There are times when uncomfortable or annoying symptoms do occur in the course of healing. In these instances, I encourage patients with a phrase commonly used in my family during moments of trial:

I am looking forward to looking back on this!

As frightening as the return of old symptoms may sound, it is my experience that it is not very much of a problem for most people. The *biggest* problem is contending with all your friends, relatives, neighbors and co-workers. On seeing you with a symptom, these sincere, well meaning people want to rush you off to the doctor, refer you to their doctor, share their

244   ✱   Everyday Miracles

prescription with you, give you medical advice and generally insist that you receive immediate treatment. They can't understand that you *are* getting treatment! Their intention is good and honorable, but this type of pressure can be enormous!

A patient of mine who had been extremely well for several years returned to see me one day saying, "I know I really don't need to be here. I just have a little cold, nothing I can't handle. It's just that the pressure at work to go to the doctor is driving me crazy! I finally agreed to come here only to satisfy them. Maybe now they'll leave me alone!" He was correct; he did not need a remedy. Sympathetic to his plight, I wrote "Penicillin" on a label and stuck it to his shirt. I told him, "I think this is what they want to see."

So few people really understand Homeopathy and what happens during Homeopathic treatment that you may find yourself somewhat isolated. On the bright side, now that you know about Homeopathy, you may find some interesting and humorous examples of Homeopathy and the misunderstanding about it in our media, culture and language.

For example, conventional doctors often refer to a dose of their medicine that won't harm patients but won't do anything to help them either, as a "Homeopathic" dose. If they only knew!

The inaccurate usage of the term even extends outside medical circles. In 1986, the securities analyst and scholar, Louis Rukeyser, noted for his insight and wit, wrote about Homeopathy in his weekly column. The article, entitled "A 1796 clue to the riddle of the U.S. policy", relates a reader's suggestion that the then current problems of inflation and deficits could be solved by applying the principles of Homeopathy.

Mr. Rukeyser writes, "Our legislators have discovered Dr. Hahnemann's theory, now that it has been abandoned by the medical people - the new interpretation being that little deficits will eventually cure a major one, and encouraging inflation will naturally extinguish inflation. The latter part of the 20th century will merely be remembered as the Age of Hahnemann Economics".

*In both these cases,
the bad news is
the information is incorrect,
the good news is
at least they have heard about Homeopathy!*

There are reasons that a remedy may stop acting other than inappropriate treatment of individual symptoms. There are some substances that act as antidotes to remedies. Homeopaths don't know exactly why this occurs, but we have consistently observed disruption of the healing process after their use. These include coffee, decaffeinated coffee, fresh mint, the drilling and Novocaine of dental work, aromatic substances including menthol, camphor, eucalyptus and moth balls. Non-therapeutic drugs such as marijuana, cocaine, LSD and heroin also stop the action of the remedy.

It is very important to avoid these substances completely. Even after many months of good health, antidoting your remedy can bring back your symptoms very quickly. It is not always so easy to correct this by just taking another dose of your remedy. In my experience, a repeat dose of remedy after an antidote doesn't work as fast or as well as the original dose. So *please* be very careful and avoid those substances during and after your Homeopathic treatment!

There are occasions when surgery or dental work is required. Alert your Homeopath first because the problem could be a return of old symptoms or other events related to your treatment. If your Homeopath decides you still need dental work or surgery, it probably will interfere with treatment. Do what is necessary and return to the Homeopath after several weeks for re-evaluation.

How long must you avoid the things on the antidote list? In a patient's language, "How long will I be deprived of my morning cup of coffee?" It takes about five to seven years for all the atoms, chemicals and cells in your body to be replaced by new ones. Therefore, the longer you are on a remedy, the more of you, the "chemical and physical" you, has been formed while in the healthier state resulting from Homeopathy. The more these positive changes are cemented in your cells, the more permanent they are and the less likely it is that you will reverse this process by disrupting your remedy. The turning point seems to be about 3 years of health. My strong recommendation, however, is always to avoid those substances.

You're probably wondering how long it will take to be restored to health. Usually, you will begin to feel better within the first month of treatment. Many of my patients state, "I feel better and stronger every day."

Curing chronic diseases typically requires one month under influence of a Homeopathic remedy for every year the symptoms have been present. This estimate also includes the time the problem was developing into its current state, not just the time that the present symptoms have been evident. Of course, all this is merely a general guideline. Other factors are the amount of conventional treatment given previously, whether any surgical operations have been performed, your overall vitality and constitution as well as your heredity, life experiences and medical history. Your specific needs must be assessed by a Homeopathic medical professional for specific recommendations and a prognosis.

One aspect of Homeopathic treatment that always amazes my patients is the short length of time they must take their remedy to gain the full benefits of treatment. Generally, only a very short course of remedy, infrequent doses or even one dose is enough treatment. How is this possible?

Once the remedy is taken, it immediately activates many of your innate healing capabilities. It is these internal mechanisms for eliminating symptoms, repairing damage and restoring health that act on a daily basis. Once this process has been set into motion by the Homeopathic remedy, no further dose is needed. It is similar to the starter on your car. A key in the ignition starts the engine, but once it is running, there are internal mechanisms in the car to keep it going. In fact, if you tried to turn the ignition while the car was already running, you could easily stall the engine. After your healing process has been started by the Homeopathic remedy, your internal mechanisms keep it going. No further dose is required. Even in treatment, Homeopathy moves you toward *freedom*. You are free from the need to take medicines for long periods of time.

How long does the good health after treatment last? Does this mean that you will never be sick again? Unfortunately, Homeopathy doesn't make us immortal. After treatment we are more resistant to adverse effects from life, but not totally immune. We live in a dynamic world of changing conditions, emotional events, relationships, growth and transition. These challenges take our energy to meet and prevail. Eventually, the wear and tear of normal living causes a slight drop in the Defense Mechanism. At this point, another dose of Homeopathic remedy is needed to restore the Defense Mechanism to its full functioning level. This may occur several months, a year

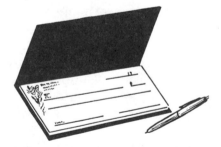

or many years after the initial treatment. There is no fixed schedule, only the symptoms dictate when to prescribe.

Think of the Homeopathic remedy as your "energy deposit", like making a deposit of money in your check book. How long your money will last depends on how many checks you write and for what amount. Infrequent small checks will make the money last a long time. Several large checks in a row will deplete the account quickly, requiring another deposit very soon.

The energy you received from your remedy also gets "used up", eventually being overcome again by the disease producing events in life. A large grief, sudden bad news and adverse living conditions are "large withdrawals" on the energy account of the remedy, making it more likely that you will require another dose sooner than if these events had not occurred. This doesn't mean that you weren't cured after the first Homeopathic remedy. It means that the dynamic qualities of life have initiated another disease again requiring Homeopathic treatment.

How will you know when it is time to get another treatment or dose of Homeopathic remedy? If you have obvious symptoms, it is clear that it is time to return to your Homeopath. My experience is that most people wait too long before recognizing that they have symptoms again. So accustomed are we to waiting until we are "really sick" before seeking treatment that people usually return to their Homeopath long after they really needed a remedy again.

Typically when we start to feel badly, tired, irritable or run down, our ever present, active minds always seem to find reasons for why we are not at our peak. "This has been a very stressful month. I've had several projects due and in the middle of all this, my car was stolen." "I know I have gotten these headaches because it has been so windy outside lately." "I'm tired but nothing is really wrong, I just haven't been getting enough sleep."

Remember, a slight decrease in the Defense Mechanism only produces minor, vague or slight symptoms.

There is really only ONE real reason
we don't feel well;
a reduction in our Defense Mechanism.

I don't tell people to return when they have symptoms. I tell them to return when they realize that they are making excuses for why they just don't feel as good as they used to.

After learning about the enormous benefits of Homeopathy, many people become very interested in Homeopathic treatment for themselves or their friends and family. I sincerely hope that this book has contributed to your greater understanding and decision to find a Homeopathy professional to treat you. A word of caution:

Not all people who call themselves Homeopaths practice Classical Homeopathy, as described by Dr. Hahnemann.

Sadly, even many who say they practice Classical Homeopathy are not following Hahnemann's method and principles. Without the strict adherence to the correct and original methods, the dramatic results that I have described are unlikely to occur. Many times improper treatment can actually cause you harm. How can you find a qualified, skilled Classical Homeopath? The following criteria will help you to maximize the chances of discovering a health practitioner that is a real Classical Homeopath. Find someone who:

1. Prescribes ONE remedy at a time.
4. Uses remedies above 30 C in strength.
3. Infrequent repetition of the dose of the remedy.
4. Uses all your symptoms to diagnose you.
5. Does not use machines to diagnose or treat you.

Giving only one remedy at a time, is an especially important aspect of proper Homeopathic treatment. There are many practitioners who violate this fundamental rule by giving several remedies at the same time, combinations of remedies or alternating remedies. This method of prescribing is not Classical Homeopathy. The only relationship it has to Homeopathy is the use of a Homeopathically prepared product.

As you recall, there are three requirements for proper Classical Homeopathy and the use of a Homeopathically prepared product is only one of the them. The others are using one remedy at a time, and prescribing by the Law of Similars. Use of more than one remedy, therefore, does not meet the basic requirements of Homeopathic treatment. It is not enough just to be taking a Homeopathic remedy, the other criteria are equally important. If you think more than one remedy can be given at a time, try singing more than one note at a time. Your vocal cords can only vibrate at one frequency at a time. You can only be in one disease state at any given time, which requires only one remedy at a time to treat.

The use of more than one remedy at a time also violates the fundamental philosophy of Homeopathy, that of the integration and unification of the whole person: mind, emotions and body. If one remedy is given for the headache, another for the pain in the elbow and still another to calm the nerves then the idea of the relationship and connection of all the symptoms representing a single disease process is ignored. This type of prescribing is following conventional medical thinking while using Homeopathic remedies.

There are many commercial Homeopathic products available that are combinations of different remedies claiming to be curative for different specific diseases. They are often labeled "headache formula", "premenstrual formula" or "hayfever formula". These products also follow conventional medical thinking, that it is possible to cure through symptomatic relief of individual symptoms. These products do not have the ability to cure the real disease that is causing the symptoms. By taking one of these products for your headache, cold, arthritis, acne or weight problem you have also lost the individuality of prescribing that is such a key element for successful Homeopathic treatment.

Often these combination products do give symptomatic relief but by doing so, they can be just as suppressive and cause just as much harm as many conventional medicines taken for symptomatic relief. The body doesn't make any distinction about what kind of treatment causes a symptom to be suppressed, if the treatment is successful in eliminating an individual symptom, then the Defense Mechanism is weakened.

One striking example of the dangers of inappropriate prescribing appeared in the June 16, 1986 issue of The New England Journal of Medicine, a highly regarded medical journal. A 34 year old man developed severe inflammation of the pancreas after taking multiple doses of a combination of 19 different Homeopathic remedies, as often as every 15 minutes, while following specific instructions from his health practitioner. He became so ill that he was hospitalized for 6 days until he recovered. Needless to say, his treatment did not follow Classical Homeopathy. This kind of irresponsible use of Homeopathic remedies should no more damage the reputation of Classical Homeopathy than should the careless use of a scalpel condemn all surgery.

The reward for Homeopathic treatment is vital, exuberant health, however, it requires responsibility and a definite commitment on your part. In this age of high speed, high pressure living with our "bottom line", "quick fix" mentality, it is often tempting to adopt that same way of treating illness. It should be evident by now that those are the very attitudes and treatments that have caused so much illness in the first place. Ignoring, covering up or suppressing symptoms instead of properly treating them from the very beginning has resulted in the chronic and serious problems so many people have today. Our options are clear. Convenience today with increasing ill health in the future, or Homeopathic treatment now with restoration of total, vibrant health.

Homeopathy may seem to have certain drawbacks for today's life style. It is even more important today than ever before because of that lifestyle. In reading his original treatise on Homeopathy, The *Organon of Medicine*, published in 1810, it is amazing to find that Hahnemann wrote about the beneficial effects of sunlight, cleanliness, exercise and wholesome foods nearly 200 years before our "enlightened" age. He even wrote about the dangers of smoking! This is especially impressive when you consider that during the era in which he lived basic sanitation was primitive at best, most peoples' diets were very poor and exercise for health reasons was virtually nonexistent. Today, Hahnemann's wisdom and insight is just as appropriate as it was when he first wrote about these things.

Why can some people exercise and change their diet and actually feel better? If what I am saying about health and disease is true, then you wouldn't expect this to occur. Let me answer this by referring back to our graph of health and disease.

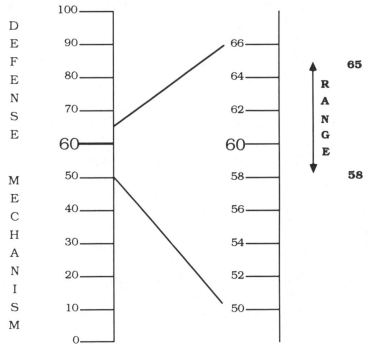

Each of us is at a specific "level", representing our health and disease activity. In this example the person is at a level of 60. There is a range of movement possible both up and down the graph. This means that we, on our own, without any Homeopathic treatment, can go from 58 to 65 and back again. This movement within the range is affected by stress levels, diet, work habits, amount of sleep and other external factors. Maintaining a proper diet, taking vitamins, exercising, positive attitudes and other active measures do, if fact, help! But the help is limited to bringing us to the top of the range in which we are confined. Since we are on a higher level of the graph, representing a healthier state, we do feel better. That is why we often think that these activities are all we need to do to restore our health. Instead of being curative, these actions are really adaptations we must make to accommodate the presence of disease.

Working diligently at nutrition, exercise and lowering stress levels must be done consistently to be of any benefit. If we stop, we will drop to the lower end of the range. Maintaining our position at the top of the range requires a lot of daily effort!

The more EFFORT, the less FREEDOM. Maximum freedom is the Healthiest state.

Doing these things or not, we are still confined to the same range on the graph. These activities, as beneficial as they are, cannot move us up and out of this range. There is always that "pull" of the disease to bring us back to the exact spot where our Defense Mechanism has determined we must be. This is why it is so difficult for many of us to do the very things that we know are good for us. Certainly, I encourage all of these good activities. They are better for us than not doing them, however, only when the disease is eliminated can we spring out of the confining barriers that restrict us to this set range.

In effect, we are better off after a Homeopathic remedy with a poor diet than maintaining an excellent diet without Homeopathy! I know this goes against almost everything you have heard and read about nutrition and health. This is because most people have only experienced the choice between being at the lower end of a range without these efforts or being at the top of that range with the efforts, while always staying in that range. They have never known what it is like to be completely above that range and in a state of great health. Many of our commonly held ideas about prevention simply don't apply to someone with a strong Defense Mechanism.

We are often told many things about what is good for our health and what is not. Whereas often these guidelines are very useful, they can be misleading. For example, how many of us have been told repeatedly that drinking eight glasses of water a day is good for us? I have heard my patients say that so often that I am sure it is a common belief. The fact of the matter is that there is no standard *right* amount of water for us to drink. We should drink what is right for us individually and our bodies will let us know how much water they want. If this sounds strange, think about watering your plants . There is no right amount of water that all plants need. You don't give the same amount to a cactus that you do to a fern. Some of us are "ferns" and some of us are "cacti".

I think the "eight glasses a day" rule must have been invented by someone who needed a remedy that had excessive thirst as a symptom. We all think that how we are is the "normal way" and right for everyone.

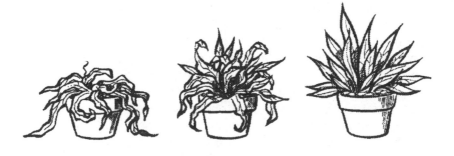

Speaking of plants, I had a plant in my back yard that just wasn't doing well. I had done all the usual "plant" things for it, but it still wouldn't grow, in fact, it had been getting much worse. I decided to put it in my neighbor's hot house so it could benefit from constant temperature and humidity, as well as protection from the elements, insects and other hazards. Once inside the protected environment, my plant started looking better and even began to grow a little. Since it was doing a bit better, I decided to bring it home. Within a week, it was drooping again. Apparently, it won't thrive in normal conditions, only in the very restricted environment of the hot house.

We all create our own "hot house" through restrictive diets, forced activities like exercise, and avoidance of normal stresses. While these efforts seem to help, they are disguising our weaknesses and they can restrict our freedom.

Avoiding exposure is not a cure.

I am reminded of so many of my patients who initially come to my office on very restricted diets because of food allergies. Yes, as long as they eat in a very particular manner, avoiding all foods containing the offending items, they feel reasonably well. These efforts mean that they can't eat in restaurants, have great difficulty traveling, are restricted at parties and other social events serving food and are limited in the variety of their own cooking and meals. Look at the price they pay to function! Although they feel better with these restrictions, as a Homeopath, I say they are still very ill because of the enormous lack of freedom.

Homeopathy strengthens your Defense Mechanism, thereby increasing your resistance, stamina and tolerance for the usual disease producing events of life. The stresses that would have bothered you in the past, now won't. Homeopathy gives you the strength to make decisions and take action to make your life better in ways you couldn't have done before treatment. Many patients report, "Normally, a week like this would have completely destroyed me, but I got through it so easily." "Suddenly it occurred to me that I was still feeling fine, even though there had been three major crises in a row." "Last year at this time, I never would have made it through the flu season without getting sick at least once. This year, I haven't had a single sick day."

Homeopathy doesn't remove life's challenges, it helps us handle them better.

The gentle, effective and deeply curative properties of Homeopathic treatment made it very popular in Hahnemann's day. This is not surprising considering the kinds of treatment available at the time: bleeding, using leeches, cathartics, the administration of crude mercury, and other toxic substances. Is this so very different in severity from the surgery and chronic dosing of medication with its resultant side effects that we use today? The permanent, thorough, safe and gentle qualities of Homeopathic treatment make it just as popular today.

Listen to some things my patients tell me during their treatment with Homeopathy: "I feel better than I've felt in years. It's been so long, I had forgotten how good it is possible to feel." "I have lot's of energy, I'm enjoying my work and I'm accomplishing things I've always wanted to do." "It's like I am really being me now. I always knew that I had this in me, but somehow, I just couldn't get it out. I just didn't feel well enough." "Words can't even begin to describe how wonderful I feel."

It is through disease that we are prevented from developing, sharing and expressing our true selves. By removing disease, Homeopathy has the ability to help you become who you really are. With the burden of illness lifted, you are given the opportunity to experience life through your true nature: healthy, free, creative and loving.

These are the

EVERYDAY   MIRACLES

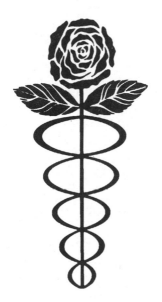

ABOUT THE AUTHOR

Linda Johnston, MD, DHt is a native of Seattle, Washington who graduated from the University of Washington School of Medicine in 1979. She moved to Los Angeles in 1980 and since that time has had a private practice in general medicine. Her practice of Homeopathy began in 1986. She is distinguished by being one of the few medical doctors in the United States who is board cerified in Homeopathy by the American Board of Homeotherapeutics.

Dr. Johnston has studied intensively with many of the most highly respected Classical Homeopaths in the world, including George Vithoulkas and Alfons Geukens, MD. She began her training with the International Foundation for Homeopathy and Hahnemann College courses and went on to study by attending many training courses and seminars in Europe over the last four years. This wide exposure has allowed Dr. Johnston to develop a deep understanding that integrates the best elements of high quality Classical Homeopathy. Her unique scholarship has lead to a remarkable book for professionals: *Repertory Additions from Kent's Lecturers on Homeopathic Materia Medica.*

To promote Homeopathy and to train professional Homeopaths, she founded the Academy for Classical Homeopathy. Currently she teaches and lectures in the United States, Canada and Europe.

Dr. Johnston is an excellent public speaker, appearing in over a hundred television, radio and print interviews. These presentations have generated an enormous amount of public interest in Homeopathy.

Academy
for
Classical Homeopathy

Linda Johnston, MD, DHt
founder and president

The Academy for Classical Homeopathy sponsors seminars and professional certification courses throughout the United States and Canada for medical professionals interested in Classical Homeopathy. Linda Johnston, MD, DHt is the featured instructor for these events. A course brochure and complete schedule are available from the Academy. (See order sheet at the back of this book.)

About Dr. Johnston:

"She helped us come to a new understanding of the material and principles necessary for the practice of homeopathy."

"You can not help but get excited and inspired"

"An excellent collection of video case histories... especially helpful"

"Information we can take back to our office and use immediately"

"A wealth of knowledge"

"You could not ask for a better teacher"

"My understanding of the use of the repertory has been expanded beyond measure"

"Amazing grasp of the materia medica and subtleties of each Homeopathic remedy"

The professional course is intended for licensed health-care professionals and teaches the methods, practice, and skills of Classical Homeopathy as developed by Samuel Hahnemann, MD. The course also relies on the teachings of James Tyler Kent, MD and modern masters in Classical Homeopathy, such as George Vithoulkas and Alfons Geukens, MD.

The study of Classical Homeopathy in all its facets and depths is a lifetime pursuit. The purpose of this course is to help you begin with a solid foundation. The curriculum is designed to emphasize the practical application of the art and science of Classical Homeopathy. Interviewing techniques, case analysis, symptom interpretation, repertory work, materia medica, observation and clinical skills are blended together in a comprehensive, innovative curriculum.

Clinical Practice of Classical Homeopathy has been developed with the assistance of an international group of recognized experts in Classical Homeopathy who have many years of experience in education and teaching. The result is a course that provides all the basic training needed to begin successfully using Classical Homeopathy.

Academy for Classical Homeopathy
7549 Louise Avenue
Van Nuys, California 91406
818-776-0078

RECOMMENDED BOOKS:

Homeopathy: Medicine of the New Man
  George Vithoulkas

The Science of Homeopathy
  George Vithoulkas

Divided Legacy, Volume three
  Harris Coulter

Lectures on Homeopathic Philosophy
  James Tyler Kent, MD

Homeopathic Medicine at Home
  Maesimund Panos, MD and Jane Heimlich

DPT: A Shot in the Dark
  Harris Coulter and Barbara Fisher

Organon of Medicine
  Samuel Hahnemann, MD

These and many other books on Homeopathy can be
obtained by mail order from:

The Minimum Price
808 Peace Portal Drive Suite AA
Blaine, Washington 98230
1-800-663-8272

Greg Cooper
Owner

RESOURCES

Academy for Classical Homeopathy
7549 Louise Avenue
Van Nuys, California 91406
818-776-0078

International Foundation for Homeopathy
2366 Eastlake Drive East #306
Seattle, Washington 98102
206-324-8230

National Center for Homeopathy
801 N. Fairfax #306
Alexandria, Virginia 22314
703-548-7790

ORDER FORM

Christine Kent Agency
17216 Saticoy #348
Van Nuys, California 91406
818-776-1881

**Please send me the following
by Linda Johnston, MD, DHt:**

Book
Everyday Miracles: Homeopathy in Action @ $17.95 _____

60 Minute Cassette Tapes

Homeopathy: An Introduction   @ $11.00 _____

Homeopathy: First Aide   @ $11.00 _____

Homeopathy for Skeptics   @ $11.00 _____

First Aid Chart (11" x 17" color)   @ $ 3.00 _____

    California residents add sales tax   _____
    Postage and handling included for tapes
    Postage and handling for <u>book only</u> @   3.00 _____

TOTAL ENCLOSED   _____

Do not send cash and allow 6 weeks for delivery.
Mastercard and Visa accepted for phone orders.

Name _____

Address _____

City _____ State _____ Zip _____

ORDER FORM

Christine Kent Agency
17216 Saticoy #348
Van Nuys, California 91406
818-776-1881

**Please send me the following
by Linda Johnston, MD, DHt:**

Book

Everyday Miracles: Homeopathy in Action @ $17.95 _____

60 Minute Cassette Tapes

Homeopathy: An Introduction   @ $11.00 _____

Homeopathy: First Aide   @ $11.00 _____

Homeopathy for Skeptics   @ $11.00 _____

First Aid Chart (11" x 17" color)   @ $ 3.00 _____

    California residents add sales tax   _____
    Postage and handling included for tapes
    Postage and handling for book only @   3.00 _____

TOTAL ENCLOSED   _____

Do not send cash and allow 6 weeks for delivery.
Mastercard and Visa accepted for phone orders.

Name _____

Address _____

City _____ State _____ Zip _____

ORDER FORM

Christine Kent Agency
17216 Saticoy #348
Van Nuys, California 91406
818-776-1881

**Please send me the following
by Linda Johnston, MD, DHt:**

Book

Everyday Miracles: Homeopathy in Action @ $17.95 _____

60 Minute Cassette Tapes

Homeopathy: An Introduction　　　　　@ $11.00 _____

Homeopathy: First Aide　　　　　　　 @ $11.00 _____

Homeopathy for Skeptics　　　　　　　@ $11.00 _____

First Aid Chart (11" x 17" color)　　　 @ $ 3.00 _____

　　　California residents add sales tax　　　　　　_____
　　　Postage and handling included for tapes
　　　Postage and handling for <u>book only</u> @　 3.00 _____

TOTAL ENCLOSED　　　　　　　　　_____

Do not send cash and allow 6 weeks for delivery.
Mastercard and Visa accepted for phone orders.

Name _____

Address _____

City _____ State _____ Zip _____